RHIA
Exam

SECRETS

Study Guide
Your Key to Exam Success

RHIA Test Review for the Registered
Health Information Administrator Exam

D1451811

Dear Future Exam Success Story:

First of all, **THANK YOU** for purchasing Mometrix study materials!

Second, congratulations! You are one of the few determined test-takers who are committed to doing whatever it takes to excel on your exam. **You have come to the right place.** We developed these study materials with one goal in mind: to deliver you the information you need in a format that's concise and easy to use.

In addition to optimizing your guide for the content of the test, we've outlined our recommended steps for breaking down the preparation process into small, attainable goals so you can make sure you stay on track.

We've also analyzed the entire test-taking process, identifying the most common pitfalls and showing how you can overcome them and be ready for any curveball the test throws you.

Standardized testing is one of the biggest obstacles on your road to success, which only increases the importance of doing well in the high-pressure, high-stakes environment of test day. Your results on this test could have a significant impact on your future, and this guide provides the information and practical advice to help you achieve your full potential on test day.

Your success is our success

We would love to hear from you! If you would like to share the story of your exam success or if you have any questions or comments in regard to our products, please contact us at **800-673-8175** or **support@mometrix.com**.

Thanks again for your business and we wish you continued success!

Sincerely,
The Mometrix Test Preparation Team

Need more help? Check out our flashcards at: <u>http://MometrixFlashcards.com/AHIMA</u>

TABLE OF CONTENTS

Introduction

Thank you for purchasing this resource! You have made the choice to prepare yourself for a test that could have a huge impact on your future, and this guide is designed to help you be fully ready for test day. Obviously, it's important to have a solid understanding of the test material, but you also need to be prepared for the unique environment and stressors of the test, so that you can perform to the best of your abilities.

For this purpose, the first section that appears in this guide is the **Secret Keys**. We've devoted countless hours to meticulously researching what works and what doesn't, and we've boiled down our findings to the five most impactful steps you can take to improve your performance on the test. We start at the beginning with study planning and move through the preparation process, all the way to the testing strategies that will help you get the most out of what you know when you're finally sitting in front of the test.

We recommend that you start preparing for your test as far in advance as possible. However, if you've bought this guide as a last-minute study resource and only have a few days before your test, we recommend that you skip over the first two Secret Keys since they address a long-term study plan.

If you struggle with **test anxiety**, we strongly encourage you to check out our recommendations for how you can overcome it. Test anxiety is a formidable foe, but it can be beaten, and we want to make sure you have the tools you need to defeat it.

Secret Key #1 – Plan Big, Study Small

There's a lot riding on your performance. If you want to ace this test, you're going to need to keep your skills sharp and the material fresh in your mind. You need a plan that lets you review everything you need to know while still fitting in your schedule. We'll break this strategy down into three categories.

Information Organization

Start with the information you already have: the official test outline. From this, you can make a complete list of all the concepts you need to cover before the test. Organize these concepts into groups that can be studied together, and create a list of any related vocabulary you need to learn so you can brush up on any difficult terms. You'll want to keep this vocabulary list handy once you actually start studying since you may need to add to it along the way.

Time Management

Once you have your set of study concepts, decide how to spread them out over the time you have left before the test. Break your study plan into small, clear goals so you have a manageable task for each day and know exactly what you're doing. Then just focus on one small step at a time. When you manage your time this way, you don't need to spend hours at a time studying. Studying a small block of content for a short period each day helps you retain information better and avoid stressing over how much you have left to do. You can relax knowing that you have a plan to cover everything in time. In order for this strategy to be effective though, you have to start studying early and stick to your schedule. Avoid the exhaustion and futility that comes from last-minute cramming!

Study Environment

The environment you study in has a big impact on your learning. Studying in a coffee shop, while probably more enjoyable, is not likely to be as fruitful as studying in a quiet room. It's important to keep distractions to a minimum. You're only planning to study for a short block of time, so make the most of it. Don't pause to check your phone or get up to find a snack. It's also important to **avoid multitasking**. Research has consistently shown that multitasking will make your studying dramatically less effective. Your study area should also be comfortable and well-lit so you don't have the distraction of straining your eyes or sitting on an uncomfortable chair.

The time of day you study is also important. You want to be rested and alert. Don't wait until just before bedtime. Study when you'll be most likely to comprehend and remember. Even better, if you know what time of day your test will be, set that time aside for study. That way your brain will be used to working on that subject at that specific time and you'll have a better chance of recalling information.

Finally, it can be helpful to team up with others who are studying for the same test. Your actual studying should be done in as isolated an environment as possible, but the work of organizing the information and setting up the study plan can be divided up. In between study sessions, you can discuss with your teammates the concepts that you're all studying and quiz each other on the details. Just be sure that your teammates are as serious about the test as you are. If you find that your study time is being replaced with social time, you might need to find a new team.

Secret Key #2 – Make Your Studying Count

You're devoting a lot of time and effort to preparing for this test, so you want to be absolutely certain it will pay off. This means doing more than just reading the content and hoping you can remember it on test day. It's important to make every minute of study count. There are two main areas you can focus on to make your studying count:

Retention

It doesn't matter how much time you study if you can't remember the material. You need to make sure you are retaining the concepts. To check your retention of the information you're learning, try recalling it at later times with minimal prompting. Try carrying around flashcards and glance at one or two from time to time or ask a friend who's also studying for the test to quiz you.

To enhance your retention, look for ways to put the information into practice so that you can apply it rather than simply recalling it. If you're using the information in practical ways, it will be much easier to remember. Similarly, it helps to solidify a concept in your mind if you're not only reading it to yourself but also explaining it to someone else. Ask a friend to let you teach them about a concept you're a little shaky on (or speak aloud to an imaginary audience if necessary). As you try to summarize, define, give examples, and answer your friend's questions, you'll understand the concepts better and they will stay with you longer. Finally, step back for a big picture view and ask yourself how each piece of information fits with the whole subject. When you link the different concepts together and see them working together as a whole, it's easier to remember the individual components.

Finally, practice showing your work on any multi-step problems, even if you're just studying. Writing out each step you take to solve a problem will help solidify the process in your mind, and you'll be more likely to remember it during the test.

Modality

Modality simply refers to the means or method by which you study. Choosing a study modality that fits your own individual learning style is crucial. No two people learn best in exactly the same way, so it's important to know your strengths and use them to your advantage.

For example, if you learn best by visualization, focus on visualizing a concept in your mind and draw an image or a diagram. Try color-coding your notes, illustrating them, or creating symbols that will trigger your mind to recall a learned concept. If you learn best by hearing or discussing information, find a study partner who learns the same way or read aloud to yourself. Think about how to put the information in your own words. Imagine that you are giving a lecture on the topic and record yourself so you can listen to it later.

For any learning style, flashcards can be helpful. Organize the information so you can take advantage of spare moments to review. Underline key words or phrases. Use different colors for different categories. Mnemonic devices (such as creating a short list in which every item starts with the same letter) can also help with retention. Find what works best for you and use it to store the information in your mind most effectively and easily.

Secret Key #3 – Practice the Right Way

Your success on test day depends not only on how many hours you put into preparing, but also on whether you prepared the right way. It's good to check along the way to see if your studying is paying off. One of the most effective ways to do this is by taking practice tests to evaluate your progress. Practice tests are useful because they show exactly where you need to improve. Every time you take a practice test, pay special attention to these three groups of questions:

- The questions you got wrong
- The questions you had to guess on, even if you guessed right
- The questions you found difficult or slow to work through

This will show you exactly what your weak areas are, and where you need to devote more study time. Ask yourself why each of these questions gave you trouble. Was it because you didn't understand the material? Was it because you didn't remember the vocabulary? Do you need more repetitions on this type of question to build speed and confidence? Dig into those questions and figure out how you can strengthen your weak areas as you go back to review the material.

Additionally, many practice tests have a section explaining the answer choices. It can be tempting to read the explanation and think that you now have a good understanding of the concept. However, an explanation likely only covers part of the question's broader context. Even if the explanation makes sense, **go back and investigate** every concept related to the question until you're positive you have a thorough understanding.

As you go along, keep in mind that the practice test is just that: practice. Memorizing these questions and answers will not be very helpful on the actual test because it is unlikely to have any of the same exact questions. If you only know the right answers to the sample questions, you won't be prepared for the real thing. **Study the concepts** until you understand them fully, and then you'll be able to answer any question that shows up on the test.

It's important to wait on the practice tests until you're ready. If you take a test on your first day of study, you may be overwhelmed by the amount of material covered and how much you need to learn. Work up to it gradually.

On test day, you'll need to be prepared for answering questions, managing your time, and using the test-taking strategies you've learned. It's a lot to balance, like a mental marathon that will have a big impact on your future. Like training for a marathon, you'll need to start slowly and work your way up. When test day arrives, you'll be ready.

Start with the strategies you've read in the first two Secret Keys—plan your course and study in the way that works best for you. If you have time, consider using multiple study resources to get different approaches to the same concepts. It can be helpful to see difficult concepts from more than one angle. Then find a good source for practice tests. Many times, the test website will suggest potential study resources or provide sample tests.

- 4 -

Practice Test Strategy

When you're ready to start taking practice tests, follow this strategy:

1. Take the first test with no time constraints and with your notes and study guide handy. Take your time and focus on applying the strategies you've learned.
2. Take the second practice test open-book as well, but set a timer and practice pacing yourself to finish in time.
3. Take any other practice tests as if it were test day. Set a timer and put away your study materials. Sit at a table or desk in a quiet room, imagine yourself at the testing center, and answer questions as quickly and accurately as possible.
4. Keep repeating step 3 on a regular basis until you run out of practice tests or it's time for the actual test. Your mind will be ready for the schedule and stress of test day, and you'll be able to focus on recalling the material you've learned.

Secret Key #4 – Pace Yourself

Once you're fully prepared for the material on the test, your biggest challenge on test day will be managing your time. Just knowing that the clock is ticking can make you panic even if you have plenty of time left. Work on pacing yourself so you can build confidence against the time constraints of the exam. Pacing is a difficult skill to master, especially in a high-pressure environment, so **practice is vital**.

Set time expectations for your pace based on how much time is available. For example, if a section has 60 questions and the time limit is 30 minutes, you know you have to average 30 seconds or less per question in order to answer them all. Although 30 seconds is the hard limit, set 25 seconds per question as your goal, so you reserve extra time to spend on harder questions. When you budget extra time for the harder questions, you no longer have any reason to stress when those questions take longer to answer.

Don't let this time expectation distract you from working through the test at a calm, steady pace, but keep it in mind so you don't spend too much time on any one question. Recognize that taking extra time on one question you don't understand may keep you from answering two that you do understand later in the test. If your time limit for a question is up and you're still not sure of the answer, mark it and move on, and come back to it later if the time and the test format allow. If the testing format doesn't allow you to return to earlier questions, just make an educated guess; then put it out of your mind and move on.

On the easier questions, be careful not to rush. It may seem wise to hurry through them so you have more time for the challenging ones, but it's not worth missing one if you know the concept and just didn't take the time to read the question fully. Work efficiently but make sure you understand the question and have looked at all of the answer choices, since more than one may seem right at first.

Even if you're paying attention to the time, you may find yourself a little behind at some point. You should speed up to get back on track, but do so wisely. Don't panic; just take a few seconds less on each question until you're caught up. Don't guess without thinking, but do look through the answer choices and eliminate any you know are wrong. If you can get down to two choices, it is often worthwhile to guess from those. Once you've chosen an answer, move on and don't dwell on any that you skipped or had to hurry through. If a question was taking too long, chances are it was one of the harder ones, so you weren't as likely to get it right anyway.

On the other hand, if you find yourself getting ahead of schedule, it may be beneficial to slow down a little. The more quickly you work, the more likely you are to make a careless mistake that will affect your score. You've budgeted time for each question, so don't be afraid to spend that time. Practice an efficient but careful pace to get the most out of the time you have.

Secret Key #5 – Have a Plan for Guessing

When you're taking the test, you may find yourself stuck on a question. Some of the answer choices seem better than others, but you don't see the one answer choice that is obviously correct. What do you do?

The scenario described above is very common, yet most test takers have not effectively prepared for it. Developing and practicing a plan for guessing may be one of the single most effective uses of your time as you get ready for the exam.

In developing your plan for guessing, there are three questions to address:

- When should you start the guessing process?
- How should you narrow down the choices?
- Which answer should you choose?

When to Start the Guessing Process

Unless your plan for guessing is to select C every time (which, despite its merits, is not what we recommend), you need to leave yourself enough time to apply your answer elimination strategies. Since you have a limited amount of time for each question, that means that if you're going to give yourself the best shot at guessing correctly, you have to decide quickly whether or not you will guess.

Of course, the best-case scenario is that you don't have to guess at all, so first, see if you can answer the question based on your knowledge of the subject and basic reasoning skills. Focus on the key words in the question and try to jog your memory of related topics. Give yourself a chance to bring the knowledge to mind, but once you realize that you don't have (or you can't access) the knowledge you need to answer the question, it's time to start the guessing process.

It's almost always better to start the guessing process too early than too late. It only takes a few seconds to remember something and answer the question from knowledge. Carefully eliminating wrong answer choices takes longer. Plus, going through the process of eliminating answer choices can actually help jog your memory.

Summary: Start the guessing process as soon as you decide that you can't answer the question based on your knowledge.

- 7 -

How to Narrow Down the Choices

The next chapter in this book (**Test-Taking Strategies**) includes a wide range of strategies for how to approach questions and how to look for answer choices to eliminate. You will definitely want to read those carefully, practice them, and figure out which ones work best for you. Here though, we're going to address a mindset rather than a particular strategy.

Your chances of guessing an answer correctly depend on how many options you are choosing from.

How many choices you have	How likely you are to guess correctly
5	20%
4	25%
3	33%
2	50%
1	100%

You can see from this chart just how valuable it is to be able to eliminate incorrect answers and make an educated guess, but there are two things that many test takers do that cause them to miss out on the benefits of guessing:

- Accidentally eliminating the correct answer
- Selecting an answer based on an impression

We'll look at the first one here, and the second one in the next section.

To avoid accidentally eliminating the correct answer, we recommend a thought exercise called **the $5 challenge**. In this challenge, you only eliminate an answer choice from contention if you are willing to bet $5 on it being wrong. Why $5? Five dollars is a small but not insignificant amount of money. It's an amount you could afford to lose but wouldn't want to throw away. And while losing $5 once might not hurt too much, doing it twenty times will set you back $100. In the same way, each small decision you make—eliminating a choice here, guessing on a question there—won't by itself impact your score very much, but when you put them all together, they can make a big difference. By holding each answer choice elimination decision to a higher standard, you can reduce the risk of accidentally eliminating the correct answer.

The $5 challenge can also be applied in a positive sense: If you are willing to bet $5 that an answer choice *is* correct, go ahead and mark it as correct.

Summary: Only eliminate an answer choice if you are willing to bet $5 that it is wrong.

Which Answer to Choose

You're taking the test. You've run into a hard question and decided you'll have to guess. You've eliminated all the answer choices you're willing to bet $5 on. Now you have to pick an answer. Why do we even need to talk about this? Why can't you just pick whichever one you feel like when the time comes?

The answer to these questions is that if you don't come into the test with a plan, you'll rely on your impression to select an answer choice, and if you do that, you risk falling into a trap. The test writers know that everyone who takes their test will be guessing on some of the questions, so they intentionally write wrong answer choices to seem plausible. You still have to pick an answer though, and if the wrong answer choices are designed to look right, how can you ever be sure that you're not falling for their trap? The best solution we've found to this dilemma is to take the decision out of your hands entirely. Here is the process we recommend:

Once you've eliminated any choices that you are confident (willing to bet $5) are wrong, select the first remaining choice as your answer.

Whether you choose to select the first remaining choice, the second, or the last, the important thing is that you use some preselected standard. Using this approach guarantees that you will not be enticed into selecting an answer choice that looks right, because you are not basing your decision on how the answer choices look.

This is not meant to make you question your knowledge. Instead, it is to help you recognize the difference between your knowledge and your impressions. There's a huge difference between thinking an answer is right because of what you know, and thinking an answer is right because it looks or sounds like it should be right.

Summary: To ensure that your selection is appropriately random, make a predetermined selection from among all answer choices you have not eliminated.

Test-Taking Strategies

This section contains a list of test-taking strategies that you may find helpful as you work through the test. By taking what you know and applying logical thought, you can maximize your chances of answering any question correctly!

It is very important to realize that every question is different and every person is different: no single strategy will work on every question, and no single strategy will work for every person. That's why we've included all of them here, so you can try them out and determine which ones work best for different types of questions and which ones work best for you.

Question Strategies

Read Carefully

Read the question and answer choices carefully. Don't miss the question because you misread the terms. You have plenty of time to read each question thoroughly and make sure you understand what is being asked. Yet a happy medium must be attained, so don't waste too much time. You must read carefully, but efficiently.

Contextual Clues

Look for contextual clues. If the question includes a word you are not familiar with, look at the immediate context for some indication of what the word might mean. Contextual clues can often give you all the information you need to decipher the meaning of an unfamiliar word. Even if you can't determine the meaning, you may be able to narrow down the possibilities enough to make a solid guess at the answer to the question.

Prefixes

If you're having trouble with a word in the question or answer choices, try dissecting it. Take advantage of every clue that the word might include. Prefixes and suffixes can be a huge help. Usually they allow you to determine a basic meaning. Pre- means before, post- means after, pro - is positive, de- is negative. From prefixes and suffixes, you can get an idea of the general meaning of the word and try to put it into context.

Hedge Words

Watch out for critical hedge words, such as *likely, may, can, sometimes, often, almost, mostly, usually, generally, rarely,* and *sometimes.* Question writers insert these hedge phrases to cover every possibility. Often an answer choice will be wrong simply because it leaves no room for exception. Be on guard for answer choices that have definitive words such as *exactly* and *always.*

Switchback Words

Stay alert for *switchbacks.* These are the words and phrases frequently used to alert you to shifts in thought. The most common switchback words are *but, although,* and *however.* Others include *nevertheless, on the other hand, even though, while, in spite of, despite, regardless of.* Switchback words are important to catch because they can change the direction of the question or an answer choice.

Face Value

When in doubt, use common sense. Accept the situation in the problem at face value. Don't read too much into it. These problems will not require you to make wild assumptions. If you have to go beyond creativity and warp time or space in order to have an answer choice fit the question, then you should move on and consider the other answer choices. These are normal problems rooted in reality. The applicable relationship or explanation may not be readily apparent, but it is there for you to figure out. Use your common sense to interpret anything that isn't clear.

Answer Choice Strategies

Answer Selection

The most thorough way to pick an answer choice is to identify and eliminate wrong answers until only one is left, then confirm it is the correct answer. Sometimes an answer choice may immediately seem right, but be careful. The test writers will usually put more than one reasonable answer choice on each question, so take a second to read all of them and make sure that the other choices are not equally obvious. As long as you have time left, it is better to read every answer choice than to pick the first one that looks right without checking the others.

Answer Choice Families

An answer choice family consists of two (in rare cases, three) answer choices that are very similar in construction and cannot all be true at the same time. If you see two answer choices that are direct opposites or parallels, one of them is usually the correct answer. For instance, if one answer choice says that quantity x increases and another either says that quantity x decreases (opposite) or says that quantity y increases (parallel), then those answer choices would fall into the same family. An answer choice that doesn't match the construction of the answer choice family is more likely to be incorrect. Most questions will not have answer choice families, but when they do appear, you should be prepared to recognize them.

Eliminate Answers

Eliminate answer choices as soon as you realize they are wrong, but make sure you consider all possibilities. If you are eliminating answer choices and realize that the last one you are left with is also wrong, don't panic. Start over and consider each choice again. There may be something you missed the first time that you will realize on the second pass.

Avoid Fact Traps

Don't be distracted by an answer choice that is factually true but doesn't answer the question. You are looking for the choice that answers the question. Stay focused on what the question is asking for so you don't accidentally pick an answer that is true but incorrect. Always go back to the question and make sure the answer choice you've selected actually answers the question and is not merely a true statement.

Extreme Statements

In general, you should avoid answers that put forth extreme actions as standard practice or proclaim controversial ideas as established fact. An answer choice that states the "process should be used in certain situations, if..." is much more likely to be correct than one that states the "process should be discontinued completely." The first is a calm rational statement and doesn't even make a definitive, uncompromising stance, using a hedge word *if* to provide wiggle room, whereas the second choice is a radical idea and far more extreme.

Benchmark

As you read through the answer choices and you come across one that seems to answer the question well, mentally select that answer choice. This is not your final answer, but it's the one that will help you evaluate the other answer choices. The one that you selected is your benchmark or standard for judging each of the other answer choices. Every other answer choice must be compared to your benchmark. That choice is correct until proven otherwise by another answer choice beating it. If you find a better answer, then that one becomes your new benchmark. Once you've decided that no other choice answers the question as well as your benchmark, you have your final answer.

Predict the Answer

Before you even start looking at the answer choices, it is often best to try to predict the answer. When you come up with the answer on your own, it is easier to avoid distractions and traps because you will know exactly what to look for. The right answer choice is unlikely to be word-for-word what you came up with, but it should be a close match. Even if you are confident that you have the right answer, you should still take the time to read each option before moving on.

General Strategies

Tough Questions

If you are stumped on a problem or it appears too hard or too difficult, don't waste time. Move on! Remember though, if you can quickly check for obviously incorrect answer choices, your chances of guessing correctly are greatly improved. Before you completely give up, at least try to knock out a couple of possible answers. Eliminate what you can and then guess at the remaining answer choices before moving on.

Check Your Work

Since you will probably not know every term listed and the answer to every question, it is important that you get credit for the ones that you do know. Don't miss any questions through careless mistakes. If at all possible, try to take a second to look back over your answer selection and make sure you've selected the correct answer choice and haven't made a costly careless mistake (such as marking an answer choice that you didn't mean to mark). This quick double check should more than pay for itself in caught mistakes for the time it costs.

Pace Yourself

It's easy to be overwhelmed when you're looking at a page full of questions; your mind is confused and full of random thoughts, and the clock is ticking down faster than you would like. Calm down and maintain the pace that you have set for yourself. Especially as you get down to the last few minutes of the test, don't let the small numbers on the clock make you panic. As long as you are on track by monitoring your pace, you are guaranteed to have time for each question.

Don't Rush

It is very easy to make errors when you are in a hurry. Maintaining a fast pace in answering questions is pointless if it makes you miss questions that you would have gotten right otherwise. Test writers like to include distracting information and wrong answers that seem right. Taking a little extra time to avoid careless mistakes can make all the difference in your test score. Find a pace that allows you to be confident in the answers that you select.

Keep Moving

Panicking will not help you pass the test, so do your best to stay calm and keep moving. Taking deep breaths and going through the answer elimination steps you practiced can help to break through a stress barrier and keep your pace.

Final Notes

The combination of a solid foundation of content knowledge and the confidence that comes from practicing your plan for applying that knowledge is the key to maximizing your performance on test day. As your foundation of content knowledge is built up and strengthened, you'll find that the strategies included in this chapter become more and more effective in helping you quickly sift through the distractions and traps of the test to isolate the correct answer.

Now it's time to move on to the test content chapters of this book, but be sure to keep your goal in mind. As you read, think about how you will be able to apply this information on the test. If you've already seen sample questions for the test and you have an idea of the question format and style, try to come up with questions of your own that you can answer based on what you're reading. This will give you valuable practice applying your knowledge in the same ways you can expect to on test day.

Good luck and good studying!

Data Content, Structure & Standards

Classification Systems

ICD-10-CM

Hierarchical structure

The hierarchical structure of ICD-10-CM is similar to ICD-9-CM in that the first 3 characters of the codes are categorized according to similar traits. The differences between the 2 editions are summarized below:

Differences	ICD-10	ICD-9
Number of Chapters	21	17
Code Structure	Alphanumeric, Length = 3-7 characters	Numeric, Length = 3-5 characters
Diseases of the Sensory Organs	Eyes/Ears separated into own chapter	Combined in the Nervous System Diseases
Injury Classification	According to site (eg, arm)	According to type (eg, wound)
Placeholder	"X" is used when a code has less than 6 characters but a 7th character is required.	None
V & E supplemental codes	Incorporated into main classification system	Available for assignment
Titles	Includes full titles for codes	Refers the coder back to common 4th and 5th digits

New features compared to ICD-9-CM

ICD-10-CM has numerous new features in comparison to ICD-9-CM, all aimed at providing a greater level of specificity and clinical detail. The new features are updated to be more consistent with modern-day clinical practices, and are as follows:

- New combination codes
- Added laterality
- Added 7th character for episode of care
- Expanded codes
- Inclusion of trimesters in obstetrical codes
- Changes in time frames for acute myocardial infarctions (8 weeks decreased to 4 weeks) and abortions versus fetal death (22 weeks decreased to 20 weeks)
- Changes in definitions of exclusion notes (e.g., Excludes1 and Excludes2)

These new features will provide data that enhances quality of care, enhances reimbursement models, improves research and clinical trial studies, and enhances the monitoring of resource usage.

Code structure

Unlike ICD-9-CM code assignments that only contained 3 to 5 characters, ICD-10-CM codes contain anywhere from 3 to 7 characters. The first character of the ICD-10-CM code will always be one of the following alphabetic letters: A-T and V-Z. Note, the letter "U" is not used because it has been reserved by the World Health Organization (WHO) for other purposes. The second character of the ICD-10-CM code will always be numeric, and the remaining characters can be either alpha or numeric. The decimal is still used after the third character in the ICD-10-CM code as it was in the ICD-9-CM code. Secondary to the expansion of the code structure up to 7 characters, there are now more than 68,000 codes, compared with only 13,000 codes in ICD-9. The expansion of the code structure allows for greater specificity and clinical detail.

Structure of alphabetic index

The ICD-10-CM alphabetic index is similarly arranged to the ICD-9-CM alphabetic index with a few differences. The following table shows the similarities and differences:

ICD Version	Index to Diseases & Injuries	Index to External Causes	Hypertension Table	Table of Drugs & Chemicals
ICD-9-CM	Yes	Yes	Yes	Yes
ICD-10-CM	Yes	Yes	No	Yes

Main terms in the ICD-10-CM alphabetic index are in bold font and vertically aligned with the left-hand margin. Indented beneath each main term are subterms with the corresponding code to be further researched in the tabular list. Only the first 4 characters of the code are listed. If additional characters are required, a dash (-) will be present at the end of the index entry. Morphology codes are no longer included in the alphabetic index for ICD-10-CM, but manifestation codes are still included in the same manner as ICD-**9**-CM.

Structure of tabular list

The key to understanding the ICD-10-CM tabular list is to be aware of how it is categorized and sub-categorized. The first principle to understand is that the list is divided into 21 chapters.

A coder must process through each available category in order to assign the code with the highest level of specificity, which for some codes will only be 3 characters, and for other codes, 7 characters. For those codes with a 7th character that explains whether it is an initial or subsequent encounter or the sequelae of a previous disease/condition, it may be necessary to use the placeholder character of "X" to fill in for any empty spaces.

A coder must process through each available category in order to assign the code with the highest level of specificity, which for some codes will only be 3 characters, and for other codes, 7 characters. For those codes with a 7th character that explains whether it is an initial or subsequent encounter or the sequelae of a previous disease/condition, it may be necessary to use the placeholder character of "X" to fill in for any empty spaces.

Instructional notes in the alphabetic index and tabular list

Instructional notes are still used in the ICD-10 books. The different types of notes are inclusion notes, exclusion notes, code first notes, use additional code notes, and cross-reference notes (e.g., *see, see also,* and *see condition*). The inclusion notes are easy to identify because they are introduced with the word "includes" at the beginning of a category, chapter, or section. Exclusion notes are divided into 2 types: *Excludes1* or *Excludes2. Excludes1* means that a code is "not coded here" or that the code should never be used simultaneously as the code above the *Excludes1* note. *Excludes2* means "not included here." In other words, the excluded condition is not part of the condition represented by the code, and, therefore, the 2 codes can be coded together if the patient has been diagnosed with both conditions. Code first and use additional code notes are similar to ICD-9 guidelines and represent underlying conditions along with their manifestations. Cross-reference notes instruct the coder to look elsewhere before assigning a code.

ICD-10-PCS codes

Major attributes

The structure of ICD-9-CM, Volume 3, for procedural coding was not capable of evolving into more codes necessary for keeping up with the explosion of technological advances in health care. It became mandatory in the ICD-10 realm for procedure codes to be designed in such a way as to accommodate growth long-term. The result was ICD-10-PCS (Procedural Coding System) with elimination of a third volume (as was used in ICD-9). ICD-10-PCS was developed with 4 major attributes and their meanings in mind: completeness (meaning – one unique code for each different procedure), expandability (meaning – ICD-10-PCS allows for the incorporation of new procedure codes), multiaxial (meaning – codes consist of independent characters with the capability of each retaining meaning across broad ranges of codes), and standardized terminology (meaning – each term must have a specific meaning). It is important that coders thoroughly understand the definitions for all the procedures and the various approaches to operations as this will be key to correct code assignments.

General principles followed when developing codes

The structure of ICD-9-CM, Volume 3, for procedural coding was not capable of evolving into more codes necessary for keeping up with the explosion of technological advances in health care. It became mandatory in the ICD-10 realm for procedure codes to be designed in such a way as to accommodate growth long-term. The result was ICD-10-PCS (Procedural Coding System) with elimination of a third volume (as was used in ICD-9). ICD-10-PCS was developed following several general principles: 1) diagnostic information is no longer included in the procedural codes; 2) there is less usage of the not otherwise specified (NOS) designation; 3) there is limited usage of the not elsewhere classified (NEC) designation; and, 4) there is expansion of the level of specificity.

Format

ICD-10-PCS is formatted in 3 sections: Tables, Index, and List of Codes. The Index is an alphabetic listing of procedures/operations. Codes are organized in the Index according to the general type of procedure. Of note, the Index only provides the first 3-4 characters of a procedural code. The remaining characters are located in the tables, and thus the tables must be referenced to assign a valid 7-digit code. The tables are designed in rows that provide options for characters 4-7 in the development of valid code combinations. The List of Codes is a comprehensive list of all procedural codes along with their descriptions. The process of assigning an ICD-10-PCS code begins with the coder accessing the Index to locate the appropriate table, and then referencing that table to locate the remaining characters for code completion.

Characters for medical and surgical procedures

Medical and surgical procedural codes are composed of 7 characters. The characters and their meanings follow. The first character represents 4 different sections: 0 – Med/Surg; 1 – Obstetrics; 2 – Placement; and, 3 – Administration. (The majority of procedural codes are categorized in the Med/Surg section.) The second character represents the body system (e.g., cardiology, respiratory). The third character represents the root operation, also known as the objective of the procedure. The fourth character represents the body part where the procedure is performed (e.g., stomach, brain). The fifth character represents the approach or method to reach the procedure site (e.g., open, percutaneous). The sixth character represents the device used during the procedure (e.g., implant). The seventh character represents the _qualifier_ that provides additional information about the procedure. Tip to memorizing the 7 characters:

Section	Sam
Body System	Baked
Root Operation	Raspberry
Body Part	Bagels
Approach	And
Device	Delicious
Qualifier	Quiche

Root operations that remove of body parts

There are 5 root operations in ICD-10-PCS that remove part or all of a body part. All 5 are done with no replacement of the body part or tissue. The 5 root operations are listed as follows (with their differences in bold):

Root Operation	Purpose of the Procedure	Site of Procedure
Excision	Cut out or off	_Portion_ of a body part
Resection	Cut out or off	_Entire_ body part
Detachment	Cut out or off	_Extremities only_; exclusive to amputations
Destruction	Eradicate/Destroy	Body part _not removed, rather destroyed_
Extraction	Pull out with force	_Portion_ of a body part _or entire_ body part

Root operations that always involve a device

There are 6 root operations in ICD-10-PCS that always involve a device. For the purposes of ICD-10-PCS coding, a device is defined as an appliance or material that remains in the body or on the body after the procedure. The 6 root operations are listed as follows (with their differences in bold):

Root Operation	Purpose of the Procedure	Example
Insertion	_Addition_ of a _non-biological_ device	Foley catheter placement
Replacement	_Addition_ of a device that _replaces_ a body part	Phacoemulsification with intraocular lens implant
Supplement	_Addition_ of a device that _reinforces_ a body part	Umbilical hernia repair with mesh
Change	_Exchange_ of a device	Tracheostomy tube exchange
Removal	_Take out_ a device	Removal of endotracheal tube
Revision	_Modification_ of a _malfunctioning_ device	Adjustment of a pacemaker lead

ICD-10-PCS coding if an intended procedure is discontinued

For example, an operative procedure is discontinued for various reasons. When this occurs, the coder must determine to what extent the procedure was conducted. Once this is determined, the coder should code the procedure to the appropriate root operation. For example, a laparoscopic cholecystectomy is planned, and the laparoscope is inserted into the abdominal cavity, but the patient becomes hypotensive and the surgery is stopped. In this case, the coder would code the laparoscopic approach only. In other instances, a root operation may not even be performed. In that case, a code should be assigned for inspection of the appropriate body part. Understanding this general guideline will aid the coder in selecting the correct root operation that represents character #3 of the procedural code.

Using the ICD-10-PCS index to locate a procedure

A coder should first reference the ICD-10-PCS index to begin the process of locating the best code for the procedure performed. The procedural codes are organized in the index based on the general type of procedure (e.g., excision, dilation, repair, removal) The index outlines the first 3 or 4 characters of a code, which the coder uses to reference the corresponding ICD-10-PCS table to complete the code. The coder must reference the table to obtain a complete and valid procedural code. The principle of referencing the ICD-10-PCS table is similar to the principle in ICD-9 coding when the coder was expected to reference the tabular list to obtain a valid code.

Layout of the ICD-10-PCS table

A coder must utilize the ICD-10-PCS table to obtain complete and valid procedural codes. The table is constructed with a top and bottom portion. The top portion of the table reflects the first 3 characters of the code (already determined from the ICD-10-PCS index). The bottom portion of the table reflects all valid combinations of code characters 4 through 7. The 4th through 7th characters must be selected from the same row of data as it expands across the 4 columns pertaining to the body part, procedural approach, device, and qualifier. It is important to understand that characters 4 through 7 cannot be selected at any place on the table; rather, the selections must remain within the same row. The options for code selections per table are innumerable.

Purpose of following outpatient coding guidelines

The Current Procedural Terminology (CPT) code set is a widely accepted nomenclature for the reporting of physician procedures and services. It is endorsed by the US Department of Health and Human Services as the nationally accepted coding standard. Each section of the CPT code book includes specific guidelines. These coding guidelines are a set of rules for coders to follow in order to appropriately interpret and report procedures and services provided in physician's offices and/or outpatient settings. As with all coding guidelines, they promote consistency among coders and healthcare providers in the assignment of codes.

CPT book

The Current Procedural Terminology (CPT) book was originally published in 1966. It is used to assign codes for procedures and/or services provided by a physician in his/her office, or provided in an outpatient setting such as a surgery center. The CPT book is published by the American Medical Association (AMA) and updated annually by a CPT editorial panel and advisory committee comprised of healthcare professionals. The CPT procedural codes are used alongside ICD-10-CM diagnostic codes on claims, and both sets of codes are analyzed by payers for reimbursement purposes. The CPT book is composed of an introduction section (instructions for using the book), 6 main sections (evaluation and management, anesthesia, surgery, radiology, pathology/laboratory, and medicine), 13 appendices (eg, modifiers, summary of add-on codes, clinical examples), Category II and III codes (supplemental and/or temporary codes), and an alphabetic index.

Assigning diagnostic code for outpatient stays

When assigning diagnostic codes for an outpatient encounter, a "principal diagnosis" would not be assigned for outpatient services because principal diagnosis refers solely to an inpatient admission. Rather, for outpatient services, the reason for the encounter or visit is called the first-listed diagnosis, or the primary diagnosis. The first-listed or primary diagnosis is determined based on the patient's presentation to the hospital. For example, when a patient presents for outpatient surgery, the coder would select the reason for the surgery as the first-listed diagnosis. This would be the case even if the surgery was canceled for any reason. In another scenario, when a patient is admitted to the hospital as an observation patient for a medical condition, the coder would select the reason for the medical condition as the first-listed diagnosis. There are times when a patient develops complications from an outpatient surgical procedure and is subsequently admitted to the hospital under observation status. In those instances, the coder would assign the primary diagnosis as the reason for the surgery followed by codes for the complications that necessitated the admission to observation status.

Specific services included in a CPT surgical code

Certain services are always bundled into the CPT surgical code in addition to the actual operation. Since the services are bundled into one CPT surgical code, they are not "unbundled," meaning they are not coded separately. The services included in the CPT code are:

- local infiltration, anesthetic block, or topical anesthesia;
- one evaluation and management (E/M) encounter on the date immediately prior to the procedure or on the date of the procedure;
- immediate postoperative care;
- physician orders;
- evaluation of the patient in the postanesthesia recovery area; and,
- typical postoperative follow-up care.

This bundled group of services can be referred to as a CPT Surgical Package.

Code modifiers

Modifiers are used quite frequently with CPT codes. Their purpose is to indicate that the procedure has been altered from the usual procedural process. With the application of modifiers, the assignment of extra separate procedure codes is avoided. Examples of when modifiers may be used are for:

- local infiltration, anesthetic block, or topical anesthesia;
- one evaluation and management (E/M) encounter on the date immediately prior to the procedure or on the date of the procedure;
- immediate postoperative care;
- physician orders;
- evaluation of the patient in the postanesthesia recovery area; and,
- typical postoperative follow-up care.

This bundled group of services can be referred to as a CPT Surgical Package.

Code symbols used in the CPT codebook

Code symbols are used in the CPT code book to facilitate quick understanding. They primarily represent additions, deletions, and revisions. A quick reference table of the symbols and their meanings are noted here:

Symbol	Meaning
Bullet	New procedure code
Triangle	Revised procedure code
Facing triangles	New and revised information in the CPT guidelines
Plus sign	Add-on code
Circle	Code has been reinstated
Circled bullets	Use of moderate sedation
Null zero	CPT codes that may not be used with modifier -51
Flash symbol	Products pending FDA approval

Importance of time in CPT code selection

Time is an important factor when considering the assignment of CPT codes. Time is understood to be the amount of time when the healthcare provider is face-to-face with the patient (e.g., evaluation and management services). It is important to understand the definition of a "unit of time." A unit of time is based on when the midpoint is passed (e.g., 31 minutes would be past the midpoint of 0 to 60 minutes). Correct time calculations in the assignment of codes for drug or hydration infusions can be challenging secondary to numerous instructions, hierarchical rules, and different payer policies. Beyond these challenges, time factors vary depending on the method of drug administration (injection, infusion, or a push). For example, a drug "injection" typically takes about 3-5 minutes to perform, whereas a drug "infusion" usually lasts for 30 minutes or more. An IV "push" is an infusion of 15 minutes or less. An initial "infusion" will be at least 16 minutes and could last up to 90 minutes. Additional hours of infusion are calculated in increments of 30 minutes. These 3 types of drug administration examples provide a clear picture of the relevance of time with CPT code selection.

Categories of E/M section of the CPT code book

The evaluation and management (E/M) section of the CPT code book is divided into general categories of office visits, hospital visits, and consultations. These categories are further subdivided into subcategories. For example, the office visit category has subcategories pertaining to new patients and established patients. Hospital visits have subcategories pertaining to initial and subsequent visits. Formatting similarities between the different categories are as follows: unique codes are listed first, followed by the place and/or type of service (eg, outpatient visit), followed by the content of the service noted (eg, problem-focused physical exam), followed by the nature of the problem (eg, the patient has developed a significant complication), and concluded with a time element associated with the service/procedure (eg, 15 minutes at the bedside).

New and established patients

To assign the correct evaluation and management (E/M) code, it is necessary to understand the difference between a new patient and an established patient, with the difference based on whether or not the patient has seen the healthcare provider within a timeframe of 3 years. In other words, if

- 21 -

a patient has received professional services (e.g., face-to-face time with a physician or even services from a physician of the exact same specialty belonging to the same group practice) within the last 3 years, then he/she is considered to be an established patient. If the patient has not received the professional services within the past 3 years (e.g., same physician practice conditions), then he/she is considered to be a new patient. These principles do not apply for a patient being seen in an emergency department.

Health Record Content & Documentation

EMR and EHR

An electronic medical record (EMR) and an electronic health record (EHR) are easily confused terms among healthcare providers, but there are differences between the 2 terms. An EHR is more comprehensive in that it contains a cumulative record of health-related information from multiple clinicians from more than 1 healthcare organization, whereas an EMR is a collection of health-related information by a single organization.

"If it isn't documented, it hasn't been done."

The statement, "If it isn't documented, it hasn't been done," has been a long-standing adage well known to health information professionals. Healthcare provider documentation of diagnoses and treatment rendered is the key to preventing denials, winning appeals, and preventing accusations of fraudulent activity by governmental agencies (e.g., Office of Inspector General, Recovery Audit Contractors). The Centers for Medicare and Medicaid Services (CMS) points out that clear and concise health information documentation is critical to the quality of patient care and is required for payment of services rendered. Documentation is necessary to support the medical necessity of services and to ensure compliance with regulatory requirements. Healthcare organizations must have policies and procedures in place to maintain the integrity of the health record.

Benefits of collecting accurate healthcare data

Benefits of capturing accurate healthcare data include: 1) improving patients' quality of care; 2) identifying disparities in the delivery of health care; 3) enhancing healthcare research; 4) identifying disease trends that aid providers in resource management and cost effectiveness; and, 5) identifying opportunities to prevent fraudulent claims submission. Accurate data assists healthcare management with fiscal planning, budgeting, development of initiatives to reduce patients' lengths of stay in the hospital as well as unnecessary readmissions, and development of methods to prevents deaths. Associations such as Healthcare Information and Management Systems Society (HIMSS) aim to optimize health through clinical informatics or data analysis. Following suit, healthcare organizations have discovered the power of data when it comes to improving quality of care; therefore, data accuracy is imperative to survival in the current healthcare realm.

Ensuring healthcare data is meaningful and useful

With healthcare initiatives focused on quality, outcomes, and payment methodologies, it is a common practice for healthcare institutions to process their data so that it is meaningful; in other words; its purpose ultimately is to promote informed decision making. For data to be meaningful, they must first be captured, queried, and finally analyzed. Data capture should ensure that all the right information is collected and stored in an appropriate format. Data queries are conducted on the collected information, but it is necessary for the data analyst to be familiar with all the systems where the data pulls from (e.g., EHR, pharmacy Pyxis systems, Chargemaster, computer-assisted

- 22 -

coding [CAC], encoders). Data analysis should include quality checks, accurate interpretation through application of statistical formulas and/or algorithms, and presentation for informed decision making.

EHR

Semantic content

An electronic health record (EHR) is a record of a patient's healthcare journey composed of electronic documents from various electronic systems. Prior to the EHR era, health information was maintained in paper records. Upon a patient's discharge, the paper records were retrieved from the hospital floors and assembled in a certain prescribed order in the HIM department. In today's EHR environment, assembly of the information means that it should be available in a logical and meaningful manner for the healthcare employee's use. Uniformity and standardization of data collection points (or fields) should be the norm. In an EHR environment, semantic content, or the inherent meaning of each data element, must retain its meaning throughout its lifetime as this promotes data integrity.

Assembly

An electronic record (EHR) is "assembled" through different means of capture: scanned paper documents, automatic feeds, and manual entry. Scanned paper documents or document imaging processes are necessary for paper documents to become a part of the EHR. Primarily, this process involves 3 steps: document preparation (e.g., removing staples, repairing tears, and organizing papers by document type), document scanning (e.g., actual physical scanning and conversion to an electronic image), and document quality control and indexing (e.g., HIM personnel check each individual image for quality and index the image based on document type). Automatic feeds of certain reports become part of an EHR, such as Admissions/Discharges/Transfers (ADT) transaction report, transcribed reports, and radiology reports. Manual entry of data by clinicians into predefined templates of the EHR is a means of data capture. Once these steps are completed, each account is processed through coding and deficiency management and finally physician authentication.

Legal health record

The legal health record is a compilation of individually identifiable data as well as the documentation of services rendered to a patient by the healthcare provider. Each healthcare entity must define in their policies and bylaws the content of the legal record. The content of the legal record may be composed of both paper and electronic documents. The content of the legal record must comply with standards set forth by external agencies, such as The Joint Commission, the Centers for Medicare and Medicaid Services (CMS), the Health Insurance Portability and Accountability Act (HIPAA), and federal and state regulations. The legal health record serves patient care, administrative, business, and financial purposes. Additionally, it is considered a legal document that is submissible as evidence in court proceedings.

ECRM

Enterprise Content and Records Management (ECRM) can be defined as the management of electronic information created and stored in analog or digital format, with the records management component referring to the creation, receipt, maintenance, use, and disposition of the health information. To manage health information/health record content at an enterprise level, various technologies, tools, and methods will be used to create, store, maintain, and deliver the health information. The life cycle of a health record is the foundation of ECRM. The life cycle begins with

- 23 -

the creation of information with the source of creation being an email, paper, or other knowledge source. The newly created health information is reviewed and edited until a final version is published via electronic health record systems, corporate portals, CD-ROMs, or PDF collections. The final version will move through a stage of active use until it becomes inactive and is retained until approved for a final disposition. ECRM tools and technologies aid healthcare entities with record management processes. These tools may include bar coding, optical character recognition, classification tools, and computer output tools to laser disks.

Unstructured data

Unstructured data are described as information that requires manipulation in order for it to be usable. Unstructured data may present itself in the form of handwritten paper notes, dictation, information contained within emails, scanned reports, diagnostic images, etc. Unstructured data are problematic for healthcare organizations because their source of origin lies in multiple disparate systems, and the majority of the data are not standardized and hard to access. Technological advances, however, are paving the way for EHR systems that are highly effective in capturing unstructured data and converting them into usable formats.

Destroying health information

Health information may be destroyed when in compliance with federal and state regulations. Destruction would be applicable to inactive records only, and the following information should never be destroyed: basic information such as admission and discharge dates, responsible physician names, diagnoses and operations, discharge summaries, operative reports, and pathology reports. Health information of minors should not be destroyed until after the period of their minority has passed plus any time pertaining to statute of limitations has passed. Disease, operative, and physician indices should be kept for a period of 5 to 10 years depending on state regulations. Birth and death certificates should be maintained permanently.

Life cycle of a health record

The life cycle of a health record is composed of 4 parts: creation, utilization, maintenance, and destruction. A record cannot exist without the creation of information; hence, the first phase in the life cycle. Creation of the health information happens for the purpose of using the information. The information collected helps to guide the healthcare practitioners in the best treatment possible for the patient through this communication tool. When an active date of service is over, the record must still be maintained per federal and state retention standards. The maintenance time frame varies depending on state regulations, but after no further treatment activity, the record is destroyed. Destruction policies and procedures must indicate the appropriate methods of destruction for each type of medium that contains the health information (eg, paper, microfilm). Electronic data would likely be archived instead of destroyed.

Potential risks associated with not having a health information retention schedule

A records retention policy is an absolute necessity in the health information field. Legal compliance with federal and state regulations pertaining to information retention establishes the framework of what information to retain and how to do so. There are risks of not having a health information retention policy, including difficulties in locating information secondary to the lack of an index, noncompliance issues related to the inability to provide information to regulatory bodies, inconsistent destruction of information in a compliant manner, and/or litigation risks. Due to these potential risks, it is important to understand how retention procedures should be done systematically and in a controlled fashion. An effective retention schedule will consider all types of

- 24 -

records created and utilized for the healthcare entity, and ensure that retention of current information and destruction of outdated information are conducted compliantly.

Expectations regarding retention of health information

The Centers for Medicare and Medicaid Services (CMS), through the Medicare Learning Network (MLN), issues news flashes regarding pertinent healthcare information. MLN Matters #SE1022 addresses medical record retention. This MLN Matters points out that state laws generally outline the retention requirements for health information, but federal laws (such as HIPAA) provide guidance as well. CMS requires Medicare providers to retain records for 10 years. CMS requires that financial records, specifically the cost report, be retained for 5 years. Not only are these requirements provided the MLN Matters #SE1022, but more detailed information can be referenced in the Code of Federal Regulations (CFR).

Data Governance

IGPHC

AHIMA's Information Governance Principles for Healthcare (IGPHC) is an organization-wide framework for healthcare entities to follow when governing information management strategies. The framework or model can be used for program development or for benchmarking. It is based on the following 8 principles:

- Accountability - An individual at the healthcare administrative level is given the responsibility of overseer of the information governance plan.
- Transparency - Information governance practices should be available for review at any time with an audit trail available to verify activities.
- Integrity - Healthcare information will meet authenticity and reliability expectations.
- Protection - Healthcare information will be protected against breaches, corruption, and loss.
- Compliance - Information governance will meet regulatory requirements.
- Availability - Information will be retrieved in a timely and efficient manner.
- Retention - Information will be retained/maintained according to legal time frame requirements.
- Disposition - Information will be appropriately disposed of, after legal time frames have passed.

Technology in the management of health information policies and procedures

Long gone are the days of 3-ring binders that housed paper policies and procedures (P&Ps). The surplus of federal and state regulations requiring healthcare entities to remain compliant demands new approaches to P&P management. Healthcare organizations must find ways to ensure their employees understand all P&Ps (which are applicable to their jobs) without mentally overwhelming the employees. Creative means to educate employees and validate their understanding is necessary in the constantly changing healthcare regulatory environment. Automated methods must be in place to disseminate information effectively and efficiently. One way to do so is to use web-based P&P management systems. As P&Ps are added, deleted, or revised, automatic email notifications with hyperlinks to the source P&P can be disbursed. These automated P&P management systems have the capability to control the policy versions and recognize duplicate and inactive policies. In addition to automated P&P management systems, online training modules, eLearning, and webinars are effective means to stay abreast of P&P changes.

Assessment of employees' comprehension of P&Ps

Just because policies and procedures (P&Ps) are made available to employees, this does not mean they understand the content and management's expectations. It is essential for management to implement measures to assess each employee's comprehension of P&Ps applicable to their job responsibilities. One way to accomplish this is to require employees to take an assessment based on each P&P. The assessments should be scored to identify areas in which lack of comprehension is evident followed by further education or training. Access to P&Ps, reading of P&Ps, and assessments pertaining to P&Ps should all be tracked or monitored. This audit trail of access and assessments can prove to an internal or external auditor that P&Ps have been applied as required by regulatory bodies.

Policies and procedures

A policy can be defined as guidance or a principle of action adopted by a governing body for the purpose of achieving a rational outcome. A policy will provide the framework or the foundation on which detailed procedures are structured. A policy is different from a law or a rule. Laws and rules either prohibit or require certain behaviors (eg, a law prohibiting being under the influence while driving an automobile; a law requiring stopping the movement of an automobile at a red light). Policies, on the other hand, merely guide one to certain actions (key word: guide). An effective policy, at a minimum, will be up-to-date, contain clearly stated outcomes that are measurable, designate accountability, be enforceable, and link to the overall direction of the organization. Procedures complement policies in that they are a sequence of steps that outline how the policy will be accomplished. It is important to note that while policies change infrequently (or possibly never), procedures change often due to many variables (eg, staffing, technology).

Key elements

Healthcare organizations should follow policy and procedure guidelines and templates and/or specified formats. The following are key elements to include in policy and procedures:

- Title (representing the subject or topic)
- Reference number for tracking purposes
- Statement of purpose
- Regulatory citations and/or external references
- Scope that defines resources
- Effective date as well as revision dates
- Administrative approval signatures
- Policy statement that identifies measurable objectives, responsible parties, and monitoring of compliance
- Detailed procedural steps.

Writing effective policies and procedures

Effective policies and procedures should be written with key essential elements. The policy statement should include measurable objectives, designation of responsibilities, and monitoring methods to ensure compliance. Policy statements are written at a broad, high level. They should be written in compliance with associated regulatory guidance to the topic at hand. Procedures outline the detailed steps for the designated responsible party to follow in order to carry out tasks. Procedural steps should list any resources and/or tools needed to follow the step. The steps should outline where the work will occur, what equates to a completed step, how communication will

- 26 -

occur between involved parties, what supportive documentation will be required, and how results will be maintained and/or stored.

Data Management & Secondary Data Sources

Uniform data collection process

The Uniform Hospital Discharge Data Set (UHDDS) was established in 1974 by the US Department of Health and Human Services (HHS) for the purpose of establishing a minimum, common core data set. The data set is abstracted at the time of hospital discharge and the following elements are mandated for reporting: personal identification, date of birth, gender, race, ethnicity, residence, hospital identification, admission/discharge dates, type of admission, attending physician identification, operating physician identification, diagnoses, procedures with dates, patient disposition, and expected payer. Each of these UHDDS elements is captured on the insurance claims form known as the UB-04. Additionally, the UHDDS coincides with the requirements set forth by HIPAA, and is the standard followed by healthcare organizations to develop ICD coding/DRG reimbursement, as well as statistical policies and procedures.

Health data standards

Data standardization can be defined as the standardization of data elements (basic units of information that are unique with distinct values). Health data should be standardized in terms of defining what data to collect, deciding how the data will be represented, and knowing how it will be transmitted across various electronic systems. In order to standardize data, certain decisions will need to be determined upfront. For example: All data elements will need to be defined; data formatting will need to be implemented so that electronic transmissions can be exchanged seamlessly; and, medical and conceptual terminologies will need to be defined.

Data mapping

Data mapping can be defined as the process of linking 2 distinct or disparate data sources for the purpose of exchanging data or information. It can be referenced as data sharing and/or interoperability. Data mapping requires frequent integrity checks or validation through continuous monitoring mechanisms or auditing processes. Accurate mapping should provide uniform, reliable, and complete data, which constitutes its integrity. Challenges of data mapping that can affect its integrity may include: drop-down pick lists, computer-assisted code assignments, templates that omit important fields, inaccurate workflows, failure to update maps, interface engines, etc. Validity testing in the production environment should be performed routinely to verify that the map is still meeting its intended purpose. Identification of inaccurate mapping results should be investigated for root cause(s) and resolved promptly.

HIM in data analysis

Demand for high-quality data translated into meaningful information is revolutionizing health care. Data collection, analysis, and interpretation processes are of paramount importance in healthcare decision making, and HIM professionals can be instrumental in assisting with or conducting these data components. To elaborate further, HIM professionals may be involved in the following 5 functional capacities: 1) data capture/collection; 2) data analysis and/or decision support; 3) distribution or dissemination of information; 4) management of health information; and, 5) information governance. HIM professionals possess knowledge and unique skills pertaining to data analytic skills, so they are valuable partners with clinical and administrative teams in healthcare operations. HIM professionals may choose to pursue the CHDA (certified health data analyst) credential that acknowledges the data analytical skill set.

Meaningful data language for data analysts to know

It is imperative to understand the language of data analytics when managing healthcare data so that it is meaningful or has value. Some of the terms are familiar, having been around for many years in the HIM world. Examples of these older terms are decision support, master patient index, national drug codes, Systemized Nomenclature of Medicine or SNOMED, and *International Classification of Diseases, Tenth Revision* (ICD-10). With the advent of new payment models, ICD-10 implementation, and new regulations to reduce healthcare spending, many new data analytical terms are becoming popular. Examples of these newer terms are data mining, data informatics, data mapping, data warehouses, descriptive statistics, information governance, interoperability, predictive analytics, blockchain, data dumpster, data scientist, medication noncompliance data, and new data flow languages such as Pig. All of these terms of data analytical language relate to approaches, systems, processes, etc. They aim to make data meaningful.

Data dictionary

A data dictionary can be defined as a tool utilized by healthcare organizations for the purpose of ensuring accurate data collection. In order for data to be reliable and usable, all users and owners of the data must understand/interpret its meaning based on the same source of truth—a data dictionary. According to a "Practice Brief" issued forth by AHIMA, "standardizing data enhances interoperability across systems," and data dictionaries promote this necessary standardization. A data dictionary should describe the meaning of each data element. For example: 1) naming conventions must match between systems; 2) definition of data elements must be explained; 3) field lengths of data elements should match between systems; 4) data types (eg, alpha, numeric) should match between systems; and, 5) data frequency (eg, monthly, annually) should match between systems. To reiterate, the primary goal of a data dictionary is to achieve standardization of data elements between various systems.

Benefits

The purpose of a data dictionary is to ensure and/or promote data integrity. It provides a clearer understanding of all data elements, aids in locating data, and promotes overall good data management. In addition to these attributes of an effective data dictionary, other benefits may include:

- Improved data quality
- Improved data reliability
- Improved data control
- Reduced duplication of data
- Data consistency
- Effective and efficient data analysis
- Better decisions secondary to better data
- Improved standardization.

Relational databases

In health care, multiple different types of data are collected: financial data, administrative data, and clinical data. The data are collected and stored in databases, with relational databases being a common type used in health care. Being knowledgeable of relational databases enhances

- 28 -

collaborative efforts between HIM and IT professionals. Input from HIM professionals pertaining to work flow, data definitions, data quality, and health information privacy/confidentiality is needed, and input from IT pertaining to relational database organization is needed to enhance collaborative discussions. Relational databases are organized into relational tables, with rows and columns of recorded data. Each field in the table describes an attribute of a record, such as a patient's last name, first name, medical record number, date of birth, etc. One table is known as a flat file. A relational database consists of 2 or more related tables that are linked to one another through a unique identifier (eg, medical record number). Through the linkage of multiple related tables, many results may be yielded that can enhance decision-making processes.

Data migration from a legacy EHR to a new EHR

Multiple steps must be considered when migrating data from a legacy EHR to a new EHR. Following are examples of best practices to definitely include in the migration:

- When negotiating talks with the vendor of the new EHR, designate in writing the expectations for the vendor concerning data migration. Part of the written agreement should address vendor transparency; in other words, identify what the vendor has accomplished in previous data migrations with other healthcare entities, and what the vendor cannot accomplish in this migration.
- Ensure that key resources are identified and available for the duration of the migration.
- Key resources will likely include representatives from HIM, IT, clinical sites, vendors for both systems (old and new), and compliance departments.
- Allow enough time to plan for the transition. Effective planning prevents missing critical steps.
- Ensure accuracy of mapping so that all data is successfully migrated.
- Repetitive testing is a necessity during the migration. Testing should identify unique elements from the legacy system that are critical for the new EHR's success.

Database maintenance

The primary purpose of database maintenance is to keep the database running smoothly. In a database, constant change occurs, meaning that information is being added, revised, moved, or deleted. It is likely that multiple people will be involved with the many changes. Because of the constant manipulation of data by multiple individuals, it is inevitable that databases will begin to malfunction. Database maintenance is necessary to identify signs of corruption, problems, malfunctioning indices, and duplicate data. One additional component of data maintenance is to search for security issues and data that have been incorrectly entered. A sign that a database may be malfunctioning is sluggish movement and/or inability to access records.

Information Protection: Access, Disclosure, Archival, Privacy & Security

Health Law

HITECH

Changes were made to the Health Insurance Portability and Accountability Act (HIPAA) in 2009 for the purpose of expanding HIPAA's coverage and strengthening protection of health information. One important change was the Health Information Technology for Economic and Clinical Health (HITECH) Act that enhanced HIPAA violation penalties. The HITECH Act is a component of the American Recovery and Reinvestment Act (ARRA) of 2009. Secondary to the HITECH Act, mandatory penalties now exist for willful neglect. These penalties can extend up to $250,000 with any repeated offenses extending to $1.5 million. The HITECH Act requires that all patients who are affected by a breach of their personal health information be notified of the breach.

PHI

Protected health information (PHI) is a common term used when discussing the HIPAA Privacy Rule. Under this Privacy Rule, PHI is defined as any verbal, written, or electronic information that identifies an individual patient. Examples of PHI are a patient's name, social security number, address, date of birth, license number, photograph, or a medical record number. De-identified information is PHI wherein the personal identifiers (examples listed above) have been removed. The de-identification process protects the patient's privacy because the remaining information cannot be directly connected to a particular patient. Once PHI has been de-identified, there are no restrictions regarding disclosure of the PHI.

Types

Protected health information comes in various forms. These forms may be paper-based, which includes faxed, printed, or copied information, or even information that has been placed in a security bin for disposal; verbal, which can be communication face-to-face or over the telephone (when communicating health information verbally, it is imperative to be aware who is nearby and keep the PHI secure from eavesdroppers); and, electronic PHI. According to HITECH, any electronic program or file that may contain PHI requires encryption, such as laptops or portable devices. Encryption converts from readable to nonreadable format. Emails must be encrypted if containing PHI. This prevents privacy violations or breaches. For ePHI, protect by logging out of a computer when away from the desk, use tough passwords, never share passwords, never remove PHI from the facility, and use computer screen privacy filters.

Covered entity

Covered entity is a common term used when discussing the HIPAA Privacy Rule. Under the Privacy Rule, a covered entity will refer to a health plan, a healthcare clearinghouse, or a healthcare provider. It is important to understand that **all** employees of a healthcare provider (e.g., a physician's office or a hospital) are considered part of the covered entity. **All** employees would include those who work in a clinical capacity (e.g., physicians, nurses, radiology technicians, laboratory technicians) and/or a non-clinical capacity (e.g., registration clerk, biller, coder, environmental specialist).

Healthcare compliance audit

Multiple types of healthcare compliance audits are being conducted in the present age. To understand the purpose of a compliance audit, one must understand the different types of audits. Hospitals should be prepared in the following areas (at a minimum) where audits are likely to occur: HIPAA, meaningful use, provider-based status, outlier payments, Medicare's Two-Midnight Rule, Inpatient Claims for Mechanical Ventilation, Ambulatory Surgery Centers Payment System, Anesthesia Services, Outpatient Rehab Services, Immunosuppressive Drug Claims, Hospice and Home Health Services, etc. The list of potential audits by external agencies is extensive. The Office of Inspector General (OIG) publishes a Work Plan for each fiscal year, and this plan is an excellent indicator of where hospitals, skilled nursing facilities, pharmacies, clinics, etc., should focus their attention for internal auditing. The purpose behind each of these external auditors essentially is to identify fraud, waste, and abuse. They are looking for opportunities to improve healthcare efficiency, and in many cases this includes holding accountable those who violate federal healthcare laws.

Governmental audits

Federal auditors have the authority to review Medicare and Medicaid claims submitted by providers. The federal government audit entities may include the Medicare Recovery Audit Contractor (RAC), Office of Inspector General (OIG), Zone Program Integrity Contractor (ZPIC), and Department of Justice (DOJ). Depending on the entity involved, the auditor will have different scopes of work, and the number of accounts reviewed, timeline of the audit, and appeals process will vary among the auditors. The RAC's goal is to reduce Medicare improper payments. The focus of the OIG, DOJ, and ZPICs is on fraud and abuse. It is imperative that healthcare organizations be prepared for governmental audits.

External audits

Hospitals experience audits from external agencies on a regular basis. The external auditors may be representatives of various federal agencies (e.g., Office of Inspector General, Department of Justice, Medicare Administrative Contractors). They may represent commercial insurers (e.g., Blue Cross/Blue Shield). The types of audits requested may pertain to charges (e.g., pharmaceutical, supplies), coding, medical necessity, fraud, etc. Complete and detailed documentation is key to proving to the external auditor that a submitted claim is valid and meets regulatory compliance.

Hospitals experience audits from external agencies on a regular basis. The external auditors may be representatives of various federal agencies (eg, Office of Inspector General, Department of Justice, Medicare Administrative Contractors). They may represent commercial insurers (eg, Blue Cross/Blue Shield). The types of audits requested may pertain to charges (eg, pharmaceutical, supplies), coding, medical necessity, fraud, contracts, policies, etc. Preparation should include the development and implementation of policies and procedures, organizational education regarding each department's responsibility during an audit, identification of individuals internally who should be involved in the audits, and determination of appeals processes.

EMTALA audit

Congress enacted the Emergency Medical Treatment and Labor Act (EMTALA) in 1986 to ensure that all people would have access to emergency services regardless of the individual's ability to pay. This Act mandates hospitals to provide stabilizing treatment for a patient with an emergency medical condition, and if unable to stabilize the patient, the hospital is required to transfer the patient to a facility where stabilization can occur. EMTALA is enforced by CMS as well as the Office of Inspector General (OIG), and either entity may conduct an audit. To prepare for an EMTALA audit, hospitals should review their EMTALA and transfer policies and procedures (P&Ps), medical staff bylaws, physician on-call lists, emergency workflows, emergency department transfer form, and emergency department signage. P&Ps should be up-to-date with EMTALA guidance. Medical staff bylaws should indicate who is allowed to perform the medical screening exam. The emergency workflow should be EMTALA compliant, and signage should be easy to understand and follow from the patient's perspective. The transfer forms must be completed in their entirety, and on-call lists must correspond with documentation in the medical record.

Healthcare compliance program

Benefits

The primary purpose of a healthcare compliance program is to establish an organizational culture that identifies unethical conduct that does not conform to federal and/or state law, payor program requirements, and/or the healthcare entity's ethical policies, and then resolves the noncompliant conduct and implements measures to prevent recurrence in the future. Compliance programs guide all employees of the health system, including the board of directors and the chief executive officer (CEO). Ethical and legal conduct must be modeled from the top down and managed through a formal compliance program. The benefits of a formal compliance program include demonstration of a commitment to ethical practices, avoidance of fraud and abuse, identification and prevention of criminal and unethical conduct, and overall improvement of the quality of patient care.

Elements

A healthcare compliance program should include, at a minimum, the following 7 elements in order to be effective: 1) written standards of conduct and established policies and procedures pertaining to expected ethical conduct; 2) designation of a chief compliance officer (CCO) who has a dual reporting structure to not only the CEO but also to the corporate compliance committee, and is responsible for operating and monitoring the compliance program; 3) Designated educational and training program for all employees; 4) compliance hotline or other means to communicate unethical behavior through anonymity; 5) systematic approach to addressing unethical behavior to include disciplinary action; 6) ongoing auditing techniques to assess compliance; and, 7) investigation and remediation of systemic problems.

High-risk areas that pose compliance problems for healthcare entities

Consistently, there are several risk areas that pose the potential for noncompliance in a healthcare institution. These areas are of a special interest to the Office of Inspector General (OIG), and may include the following: billing for services never performed; providing medically unnecessary procedures or services; duplicate billing; upcoding; unbundling; violation of the patient's freedom of choice related to post-hospital care (eg, home health, rehab); violation of the Stark Law; inaccurate or false cost reporting to federal payers; violation of the anti-kickback statute; and DRG assignments that provide a higher reimbursement rate than accurately reflected in the documentation ("DRG creep"). This is not an exhaustive list; there may be other areas of high risk depending on the healthcare entity. Each healthcare entity should perform risk assessments annually in preparation of audit planning. Risk assessment functions include interviewing management throughout the healthcare system for the purpose of gleaning information pertaining to those areas where risk of noncompliance is evident.

Data Privacy, Confidentiality, and Security

Using aliases for PHI protection

Inevitably, in health care, situations will arise wherein a patient's health information may need full identity restriction. Full identity restriction may be necessary for those patients whose health information is more sensitive, especially during episodes of active care. Examples may include celebrities, politicians, athletes, victims of crime or violence, child/adult abuse, and/or prisoners. Any patient should be provided the opportunity to request anonymity or the use of an alias. It is necessary for healthcare entities to develop policies and procedures (P&Ps) pertaining to aliases as well as patient alias documentation forms. P&Ps should address when an alias can be used and how its use will affect continued patient care in future admissions. The P&Ps should ensure that all components of the EHR are linked with the alias name. The alias documentation form should include the following elements, at a minimum:

- Patient's legal name
- Patient's alias name
- Medical record number
- Staff completing the alias form
- Requestor's name (e.g., patient, power of attorney)
- Reason for the request
- Department notifications.

Policy and procedure considerations for privacy of health information

In today's healthcare environment, HIPAA compliance pertaining to security and privacy is a legal requirement. Healthcare entities are tasked with developing policies and procedures (P&Ps) pertaining to privacy. Following are considerations for the development of privacy P&Ps, all to be validated by legal counsel:

- Review existing P&Ps to determine where additional information is needed or changes are necessary.
- Develop an oversight committee of key individuals (eg, legal, HIM, privacy officer, compliance) to review the existing P&Ps and the development of new P&Ps.
- Develop a catalog or index (paper or electronic) of all P&Ps to manage the development and revision of the documents.
- Privacy topics to incorporate into the P&Ps should include the Notice of Privacy Practices, business associates' responsibilities in relation to privacy, handling of privacy breaches, investigation processes for privacy breaches, requirements for "meaningful use" protection of patient health information (PHI), how to manage patient consent for release of information, and how to manage access and disclosure of PHI.

Securing health information

Part of the Health Insurance Portability and Accountability Act (HIPAA) addresses the Security Rule. In order for providers to comply with HIPAA's Security Rule, a risk analysis must be conducted in order to identify and implement measures to ensure the security of electronic protected health information (e-PHI). The primary purpose of the risk analysis tool is to thoroughly assess potential risks and vulnerabilities to the privacy, integrity, and accessibility of a provider's e-PHI. For identified risks and vulnerabilities, a provider must initiate a risk management process. The best practice a provider can follow is to implement an integrated risk analysis and management process that is a continuous process that assesses new technologies and operations as they are initiated.

Review Video: Confidentiality
Visit mometrix.com/academy and enter code: 250384

Administrative, physical, and clinical safeguards for PHI

Protected health information (PHI) must be protected by administrative, physical, and technical safeguards. Administrative safeguards refer to policies and procedures that address PHI security as well as a security risk assessment and risk management plans. Physical safeguards can be in the form of facility access controls to information technology (IT) areas (eg, badge-only access), restrictions of computer station access, use, and security, and hardware and media controls (eg, how to properly dispose of IT media, how to back up IT media). Technical safeguards are safeguards that are integrated into IT systems to protect access to IT data. For example, individual authentication ensures the person needing access is a valid requestor.

Passcodes

Passcodes or passwords are the simplest form of security for protected health information (PHI). However, they can be the easiest to crack by those with the wrong intentions. Maintaining passcodes can be frustrating for the user due to the many different passcode requirements for different systems. Healthcare entities should have effective policies and procedures (P&Ps) in place to address the requirements for passcodes. The P&Ps should incorporate at a minimum the following points to prevent passcode cracking:

- Avoid use of words written backwards.
- Avoid use of personal information.
- Use passcodes with long lengths, complex width (meaning use of symbols, and not primarily alpha characters), and complex depth (e.g., passcodes that are not easily guessed).
- Use encryption.
- Instead of writing down passcodes, write down phrases to jog the memory of the passcode.
- Change passcodes on a frequent basis.
- Lock accounts with more than 3 unsuccessful attempts.

Developing strong passcodes

Passcodes are one essential way to secure protected health information (PHI). They are not foolproof, however, to hackers. Following are key tips regarding strong passcodes:

- Create passwords that cannot be easily guessed.
- Change passwords frequently.
- Do not use the same password for multiple systems.
- Use a combination of capitalization, symbols, numbers, and alpha characters.
- Do not always capitalize the first letter of the passcode; rather, capitalize an alpha character in the middle or at the end of the passcode.
- Never use part of the username as part of the password.
- Use a word in its numerical equivalent of a telephone pad (eg, flash would convert to 35274).
- Use 2 words separated by symbols.
- Use the first letter of each word in a phrase (eg, I love McDonald's tea becomes ILMT).

PHI breaches

Protected health information breaches are those actions in which the information is released or disclosed inappropriately and which result in a violation. A breach can even be conducted out of concern or curiosity. Common types of PHI breaches are as follows: 1) Accessing personal records. One does have the right to view his/her own personal records, but he/she must go through appropriate channels according to the organization's policy. 2) Accessing family records. This can only occur when caring for a family member in a professional capacity. 3) Friends/coworkers. This can only occur when caring for a friend/coworker in a professional capacity. 4) Celebrities. This can only occur when caring for the celebrity in a professional capacity.

Breach of confidentiality

A healthcare privacy breach or breach of confidentiality is an inappropriate or impermissible use or disclosure of health information. This type of breach is a direct violation of the Health Insurance and Portability and Accountability Act (HIPAA), also known as the Privacy Rule. A breach may occur when the security or privacy of the protected health information (PHI) is compromised. If the covered entity, responsible for the breach, can demonstrate that the PHI was not viewed or that the entity has taken steps to mitigate the risk, the release may not be considered a breach. There are other exceptions to the definition of breach, which may be described as: 1) an unintentional acquisition made in good faith, 2) an inadvertent disclosure between healthcare entities, or 3) a situation wherein the recipient of the PHI did not retain the information.

Reporting privacy violations internally

When an employee suspects a privacy violation, he/she should immediately alert his/her manager. If this is not an appropriate option (e.g., the manager may be the violator), the privacy officer and/or corporate compliance officer (CCO) should be notified through email or by calling the healthcare entity's employee Compliance Hotline. An option to report a suspected privacy violation anonymously must be made available to employees, such as a Compliance Hotline. CCOs or privacy officers will investigate further the suspected violations through interviews, interrogations, and computer analysis. The determination to proceed with seeking the advice of legal counsel will be made, and reporting of violations may be necessary depending on the severity of the violation. Disciplinary action, up to and including termination of the violator's employment, may be an appropriate course of action.

Reporting healthcare privacy violations to regulatory bodies

Anyone can file a privacy or security violation complaint with the Office for Civil Rights (OCR). The complainant, as mentioned, can be anyone, such as healthcare employee who works for the entity where the violation has allegedly occurred, or someone not affiliated with the healthcare entity. The complaint can be filed in writing, via fax, through email, or via the OCR portal. When filing the complaint, the following information should be provided: name of the complainant, contact information, and details of the suspected violation. After receiving the complaint, the OCR will investigate further and will only take action if they determine that rights were violated and the complaint was filed within 180 days of its occurrence. The OCR will issue a letter describing their investigation and they may issue corrective action for the healthcare entity or impose civil monetary penalties.

Penalties associated with healthcare privacy violations

The American Recovery and Reinvestment Act of 2009 established the civil penalties associated with healthcare privacy violations of Health Insurance Portability and Accountability Act (HIPAA). The penalties can be as follows:

Violation	Minimum Penalty	Maximum Penalty
Unintentional disclosure of PHI	$100 *per* violation up to $25,000 annually for repeat violations	$50,000 *per* violation up to $1.5 million annually
Reasonable cause, not due to intentional neglect	$1,000 *per* violation up to $100,000 for repeat violations	$50,000 *per* violation up to $1.5 million annually
Due to intentional neglect but violation corrected	$10,000 *per* violation up to $250,000 for repeat violations	$50,000 *per* violation up to $1.5 million annually
Due to intentional neglect and violation not corrected	$50,000 *per* violation up to $1.5 million annually	$50,000 *per* violation up to $1.5 million annually

Use of data mining to improve release of information processes

Privacy officers and HIM directors should routinely collaborate to analyze PHI breaches. It is important to drill down into the release of information data for 2 reasons: determine why a breach happened, and prevent future incidents of improper releases. Release of information (ROI) data to be collected at a minimum should be: documentation type improperly released (eg, discharge summary, progress notes), discovery date, hospital or clinic responsible for improper release (for healthcare systems), disclosure type (eg, misdirected fax, HIPAA privacy), release of information staff, and patient name. Audits of ROI logs should be the source of truth when digging deeper into the privacy violations. Once the root causes are identified, education and ongoing assessment should be conducted, all for the purpose of mitigating risks of future errors and improving the ROI staff's work performance.

Release of Information

Disclosure

Disclosure can be defined as the act of sharing information. In terms of the Health Insurance Portability and Accountability Act (HIPAA), disclosure may mean protected health information (PHI) has been released or transferred, or access to the PHI has been granted to a party outside of the organization who owns the information. The disclosure may happen in one of two ways: It is either an authorized disclosure or an unauthorized disclosure. An unauthorized disclosure comes with consequences or penalties.

Medical record request process

Health information must be kept confidential, and the healthcare world is regulated by laws and policies which require confidentiality. In order to access patient information, healthcare institutions must follow release of information processes to ensure privacy is protected. An authorization to disclose personal health information (PHI) form must be submitted to the health information management (HIM) department. The form must be completed in its entirety and must designate specifically which records to release. Requestors must present government-issued photo IDs in order to validate the release. In addition to this process, healthcare institutions are providing to patients the option of accessing their PHI through web-based portals. This can provide faster access to PHI instead of waiting up to 30 days for a release through other mediums (CDs, DVDs, paper).

Confidentiality in physician-patient relationship

The physician-patient relationship is considered to be a contractual agreement. The patient seeks out the services of a physician, and the physician accepts the patient for treatment. During this relationship, health information is gathered and exchanged between the 2 parties. Trust between the physician and patient is essential for the sharing of sensitive health information. Without trust in the relationship, confidentiality would be undermined. The principle of confidentiality requires physicians to keep all patients' health information private. When a patient understands his/her information will be kept private, he/she will be encouraged to seek out care and be open during the visit about his/her health condition. This is especially important with information pertaining to diseases of psychiatric, sexual, and/or drug/alcohol origins.

Written authorization to release information

When a patient requests release of his/her health information to himself/herself or a third party, a written authorization is required. A written authorization to release information should include the following components:

- Name of the healthcare entity releasing the information
- Name of the individual to receive the information
- Patient's full name and other identifying data (eg, address, date of birth)
- Purpose for needing the information
- Type of information to be released with specified dates of service (eg, discharge summary, operative report)
- Authorization expiration date
- Authorization revocation statement
- Patient's or legal representative's signature and date.

Prohibition of re-disclosure

When a healthcare entity releases patient information to a third party, a statement should be included in the release that prohibits re-disclosure. Once the health information is released, the releasing healthcare entity has no control over what happens to the information from that point forward. It is necessary for the releasing healthcare entity to include a statement that prohibits re-disclosure. This statement informs the recipient of their obligation in maintaining privacy of the patient's health information. The statement should instruct the recipient to only use the information for the intended purpose noted in the release.

Privacy Rule and disclosures of PHI

The HIPAA Privacy Rule was passed in 2003 for the purpose of ensuring the privacy and security of protected health information. The standards enforced by the Privacy Rule pertaining specifically to disclosures are as follows: Disclosures requiring authorization are identified (eg, subpoenas, court orders). Individuals eligible to authorize disclosures are noted. Examples may include power of attorney, legal guardian, or permission by a physician in psychiatric cases. Minimum necessary standards are established to limit the amount of information disclosed. Proper disclosures to individuals involved in the care of the patient are designated (eg, nurses, physicians, therapists).

Requirements for de-identification of health information for disclosures not requiring an authorization are designated. An example of when de-identification is required would be when a coding case is submitted to 3M Nosology for coding advice. In this scenario, disclosure of PHI is forbidden by the third-party vendor. The only way to receive coding feedback is to de-identify the submitted case.

Informatics, Analytics & Data Use

Health Information Technologies

HIM technology concepts and terms

In today's health information environment, technology applications are abundant. Migrations from paper-based record systems to electronic health records are the norm in healthcare entities across the nation. With the transition to electronic-based systems, new terminology and concepts were developed, with the commonly known terms/concepts affecting HIM applications as follows. Operating systems are the software programs that provide the infrastructure of interactions between applications and the computer hardware. Microsoft Windows, Mac, and Linux are examples of operating systems. Web applications are increasingly popular in healthcare operations. Common programming languages, such as C++, Java, Net frameworks, and Citrix, are widely used throughout health care. Use of natural language processing (NLP) tools are expanding in HIM operations, especially concerning coding processes. NLP is built into computer-assisted coding (CAC) functions, which enhances the coding process. Networks, such as virtual private networks (VPN) or SaaS (software as a service) and/or cloud computing, are shifting electronic functionalities from individual computers to internet-based networking.

Functional reality of software applications

To implement and manage software applications effectively, it is important for HIM professionals to understand how software programs/applications are designed and developed first. The best software programs/applications will be conceived, designed, and developed by those who have hands-on experience in the related field. After an idea is conceived, the next step is to design the concept from a functional and technical design perspective. This is followed by a technical build that is then tested for appropriateness of functionality. Rollout of the software occurs next via a beta release, followed by the general release, and then any patches to fix software glitches are implemented as needed.

Evaluation of HIM software applications

Choosing the best hardware or software application for an HIM function requires extensive investigative work beforehand. A recommended list of criteria to evaluate hardware or software follows:

- Determine what the hardware/software needs to accomplish. Be careful to not be distracted by "bells and whistles," but rather focus on the overall objective(s) that the hardware/software application needs to address.
- Determine its usability. Is it user friendly?
- Determine not only the purchase cost, but also the maintenance fees and upgrade costs.
- Seek out the opinion of other users of the proposed application. These unbiased opinions can be extremely instrumental in helping to make the best choice.
- Determine the support system for the product. Is technological assistance available 24/7 via a toll-free phone line or online service? Does support cease after the initial training?
- Determine the flexibility of services associated with the product. Are there options or services that can expand the use of the application in the future?

- Determine the level of security and privacy built into the product.
- Determine user interface capabilities. This may require the assistance of IT professionals to ask pertinent interface questions.

Initial market research when selecting hardware/software programs/applications

The process of hardware/software selection may be approached in a variety of ways. One recommended method is to conduct initial market research. Initial market research may simply mean communication with other users of the proposed product to glean their opinion. A best practice would be to organize a selection team of experts to evaluate and select the best product. This eliminates a single-person perspective or bias, providing more of a collaborative effort in the selection process. The selection team may want to pursue the following steps when conducting initial market research activities:

- Distribute vendor surveys to solicit proposals.
- Request vendor white papers, which provide detailed descriptions of their product(s) and/or case studies.
- Request technical specifications pertaining to the product(s).
- Seek input from multiple vendors at technology conferences.
- Conduct a pre-bid conference with potential vendors (or individually scheduled meetings and/or demos) to discuss the healthcare entity's needs and the vendors' proposal(s) to meet the need(s).

Information Management Strategic Planning

Data presentation

Data alone do not necessarily tell a story or show trends or even suggest successes or failures. Compiling and then analyzing data is one step in the right direction towards providing insight into successes and/or failures and subsequently assisting in making decisions. After the data have been synthesized, the next step is to present the information, usually to management or administration. Excel is an excellent tool that can extract significance from big data, specifically through Pivot table functionality. Charts and graphs can subsequently be generated from Pivot table functions and then linked into PowerPoint presentations or SharePoint Dashboards. When creating the visual presentations, determine the main objective that needs to be represented to the viewer. There should always be a singular point to make about each slide so that the viewer's comprehension or insight into the data's meaning will be quickly attained. Techniques to effectively communicate the meaning of data include: simplify the focus; be methodical and clear with the data presentation; eliminate distractions; choose the type of chart/graph that is impactful to the viewer (e.g., bar, pie, line graphs); replace text with visuals.

Presenting coding compliance audit data to administration

In healthcare entities, coding compliance audit data pertaining to accuracy, productivity, and net financial impact will be of interest to its administration on a quarterly basis. PowerPoint slides representing these 3 components are best displayed as follows: Use visual graphs rather than words to communicate pertinent information. For coding accuracy, use trending bar graphs instead of stacked columns or pie charts. Trending bar graphs will provide the administration with a snapshot of how accuracy rates fluctuate from month to month. The trending bar graph should include the expected benchmark standard (eg, 95%) graph line as well as inpatient and outpatient coding accuracy rates that may trend above or below the benchmark percentage. For productivity

- 40 -

rates, trending should be used with explanations included as to any decrease in volume (eg, vacations, training, vacancies). The net financial impact should be represented from 2 perspectives: The current quarterly monetary value (positive or negative) and the year-to-date monetary value. These 3 components of coding compliance audit activities may be used for other purposes, such as cost benefit analyses, cost justification for additional staff, etc.

Analytics & Decision Support

Providing decision support to clinicians

Secondary to the immediate availability of clinical information through electronic health records, decision support services are more timely than ever. Providing these services to a clinician should be carried out via the following measures:

- Upon receipt of a request for clinical information, the request should be evaluated, prioritized, and resources allocated.
- Research of evidence-based and best practices should occur to build knowledge.
- Analysis of the current situation should occur to understand the problem in depth.
- Design solutions for testing or piloting purposes.
- Implement solutions once design improvements are achieved.

Decision support services can be instrumental in evidence-based care but only if the clinician's needs are thoroughly understood.

Filtering data

Filtering data is a temporary solution to hide unwanted data. Through the filtering process, large quantities of complex data are reduced to smaller volumes. This simplifies the data analysis process because it eliminates redundant, irrelevant, or useless information. If filtering is not conducted, then the reviewer of the data can become overwhelmed at the magnitude of information, and thus may not be able to make accurate and reliable decisions. Data filtering may be used for the purpose of hiding or removing sensitive or private information. In health care, this may mean that personally identifiable information, such as patient names, social security numbers, or account numbers, are not included in the end result made available to multiple readers. Data filtering can be used as an extra layer of security protecting patients' health information.

Informatics, Analytics & Data Use

Healthcare stakeholders

Healthcare stakeholders are individuals or groups of people who have a vested interest in a healthcare decision. These individuals/groups may be the patients, the clinicians, researchers, professional associations, board of trustees, third-party payers, or even federal/state policymakers. Each stakeholder is interested in healthcare activities from different important perspectives. For example, patients may be interested in the aspects of an illness that are concerning. Clinicians may be interested in reliable data that will impact their medical decision-making activities. Policymakers may be interested in valid data that will support policy (e.g., national coverage determinations) revisions or policy development. Each stakeholder, regardless of perspective, will be affected by decisions made or courses of action implemented, and either the stakeholder will gain or lose something in the process. The reality of gain or loss enforces the importance of their perspective.

Data mining

In order to retrieve medical record or health information data, it is beneficial for a healthcare provider to implement a robust data mining program. For data mining to yield reliable results, the best practice would be for a healthcare entity to have all electronic systems and/or applications (with data collection) interfaced. Unfortunately, this concept is not a reality for healthcare providers, but progress toward that end is being achieved. In the interim, healthcare providers should be knowledgeable of all their electronic systems, the data housed therein, and the means of gathering and reporting from all the systems. Revenue integrity data mining systems can be purchased or even built internally to maintain/manage data. Effective filtering processes can be highly effective in yielding meaningful results.

Database query

Simply put, a database query is a request for information. Before a query can be submitted, the database must be designed using data, tables, and relationships between the tables. Once completed, select queries can be created. It is important to remember that queries can only be written in the language the database requires, which is usually structure query language (SQL). SQL is a popular choice for queries and is capable of advanced query processes. The select queries will search and find requested information from each appropriate corresponding table and then extract the information into a datasheet. The end result is called a record set, and these record sets can then be translated into reports or forms, or used for other queries.

Healthcare Statistics

Percentages

Percentages are widely used in healthcare statistics. It is essential to know how to compute percentages. A percentage is defined as the whole divided into 100 parts. A percentage can be misleading to organizational stakeholders if the total volume (or whole) is 20 or less. It may be necessary to report only when the volume is more than 20, which may mean quarterly or annual reporting. A percentage can be computed when a fraction is converted into units of 100. For example, if the fraction is 3/4, then the percentage is computed by dividing 3 by 4, resulting in a decimal of 0.75, which is then converted into a percentage by moving the decimal 2 places to the right and adding the percent sign (%). For decimal results that are lengthy (eg, more than 2 decimal places), the healthcare entity/department should have a policy that designates the number of decimal places to round to (eg, 21.456% would round to 21.5%). Once a percentage is calculated, it may be referred to as a rate. In health information management (HIM) practices, rates are a common calculation, such as death rates, birth rates, readmission rates, etc. It is important to ensure that percent calculations are computed correctly, as it can be easy to misrepresent the true picture.

Mortality rates

Death rates, also known as mortality rates, are important information in health care as they can represent the quality of health services. Death rates are represented in percentages and represent the number of inpatient hospitalizations that ended in death. DOA (dead on arrival) cases, abortions (whether therapeutic or spontaneous), and patients who die in the emergency department (without an order for admission to the hospital) are not included in the rate. Various death rates can be calculated: gross death rate (number of deaths of inpatients in a period/number of discharges [including deaths] in the same period), net death rate (formula: total number of deaths of inpatients minus deaths occurring less than 48 hours from admission x 100/total number of discharges [including deaths] minus deaths occurring less than 48 hours from admission), anesthesia death rate (defined as a death occurring while the patient is under anesthesia or caused by anesthetic agents), postoperative death rate (defined as deaths occurring within 10 days after surgery), maternal death rate, and neonatal death rate.

Length of stay calculations

Length of stay refers to the number of days a patient is designated as an inpatient from the date of admission until the date of discharge. This calculation is monitored daily by healthcare entities because it helps to evaluate and manage hospital resources. To compute the length of stay, the date of admission is subtracted from the date of discharge. For example, if a patient was admission on February 2nd and then discharged on February 9th, the length of stay would be 7 days. If the patient is admitted and discharged the same day, the length of stay is counted as 1 day. The average length of stay (ALOS) is a rate consistently monitored by healthcare entities. The ALOS rate is calculated by dividing the total length of stay (also known as discharge days) by the total discharges. For example, 1,500 patients were discharges during the month of February. The combined length of stay for these patients was 7,552 days. The ALOS rate would be calculated as follows: 7,552/1,500 = 5.03 or rounded to 5 days.

Measures of central tendency

In statistical analysis, central tendency is known as a single measure that determines the center or middle value of a data set. The 3 measures of central tendency are the mean, median, and mode. HIM professional should be familiar with these 3 measures as they are commonly used in healthcare statistics. The mean is the average of numerical values in a data set. To calculate the mean, the numerical values are summed and then divided by the number of values in the data set. For example, the mean of 2 + 3 + 6 + 4 = 15/4 = 3.75. The median is the center value in a distribution list. For example, the median of 1, 2, 3, 4, and 5 is 3 because 50% of the values lie before it and 50% after it in the distribution. The mode is the value that occurs most frequently in the data set. For example, the mode of 1, 1, 2, 3, 4, and 5, would be 1 because it is present more than in any other number in the data set.

Analyzing data to reduce readmission rates

Readmission of patients within 30 days, or even up to 90 days, can be costly to a healthcare system. Studies show that readmission costs can range between 60% and 135% of the initial hospitalization. Healthcare entities are quite interested in methods to reduce readmission rates. Many entities will implement data analytic strategies to aid in reducing the readmissions. There are models that are capable of predicting the probability of a patient's readmission potential based on their disease process. With such predictability models, clinicians can design discharge programs that will prevent readmissions. EHRs (and the abundance of health information contained within them) support the prediction models and help analysts to systematically identify methods of prevention.

Research Methods

Credibility of a source

The volume of healthcare data available through various means (e.g., Internet, journals) can be overwhelming, especially when determining which sources are credible. Information contained within professional journals tend to always have identifiable sources and authors, and are more reliable than Internet sources that need to be investigated more extensively for credibility. Guidance on how to best determine the credibility of a source includes the following tips:

- Credible sources will be those for which there is no hidden motive, and the information is presented as fair and objective.
- The author will be a subject matter expert or will have the required experience necessary to speak about the topic.
- Peer review of a publication adds support to the credibility.
- Published contact information by the publisher and/or author lends to its legitimacy.
- A web address ending in .gov or .edu tends to be a reliable source.
- Information from a randomized controlled study will be a credible source.
- The information will be cited.

Consumer Informatics

Informatics

Informatics can be defined as the applied science of data processing and information management. Informatics is used extensively in healthcare to analyze data for multiple purposes, such as strategic planning, evaluation of disease management, clinical decision support, evaluation of treatment effectiveness, and identification of potential adverse drug reactions prior to drug administration to the patient. Healthcare administration relies on clinical informatics to assess patient case mix, disease trends, compliance risks, bed utilization efficiency, and research-related foci pertaining to medication trials, medical device trials, and clinical trials. Trending of data generated through informatic tools is essential to forecasting the future of a healthcare enterprise, thus validating the vital importance of informatics in health care.

Patient health portal

The overall purpose of a patient health portal is to improve patient outcomes. A patient health portal is a secure online website that allows patients to access their health information at any time of the day from anywhere via an Internet connection. Through the portal, patients are able to view

- 44 -

various types of health information, such as medications, allergies, lab results, and physician notes. Patients may be able to communicate with healthcare professionals regarding rescheduling of appointments and requesting of prescription refills. Patient health portal access is expected to continue to grow in the coming years, and educational efforts to encourage more patients to use this avenue of communication should be pursued.

Common concerns

The overall purpose of a patient health portal is to improve patient outcomes. Along with new technological approaches to healthcare, there are concerns related to patient health portals such as:

- Healthcare providers will be overwhelmed with electronic communications (eg, emails). The opposite has happened with implementation. Providers have reported increased communication efficiency and have not been inundated with emails.
- Patient will incorrectly use the messaging options through the portal. Studies have been conducted pertaining to patient messaging through the portal, and it has been determined the message content has been appropriate. Patient education is key to understanding appropriate ways to use the messaging option.
- Providers will not be able to bill for time used addressing patient's questions and concerns submitted through the portal, and thus loss of revenue will happen. Studies show that cost savings have occurred through portal use because labor costs are reduced, telephone time is reduced, and scheduled methods have been improved.
- Patients will be unable to adapt to portal usage. Studies show that patients prefer using portals over communicating directly with providers.

Information excluded from portal access

Healthcare entities should develop policies regarding the types of information to be excluded from portal access. These decisions should comply with federal and state regulations. The following types of information should be considered for exclusion: behavioral health, minors, research, business, and other sensitive information. Behavioral health information is protected by state law, and providers may choose to deny access to behavioral or psychiatric information if they feel it could potentially harm a patient's mental health state. Information pertaining to minors is protected by state law, and the protection varies from state to state. It may be permissible for a parent or guardian to sign up as a proxy and be able to access the minor's information, but any protected information should not be available for review. Research information should not be accessed via a portal because the knowledge the patient obtains from reading the research plan (e.g., placebo use instead of actual drug use) could be detrimental to the study's success. Business information should not be made available through portal access because the information is not related to actual treatment/care. It may be decided that other sensitive information should not be accessible for various reasons, such as clinical photography, genetic testing, or HIV results.

Implementation in a healthcare entity

When considering implementation of a patient portal system, a committee of stakeholders should be organized to manage the overall selection and implementation process. The committee should identify the primary functionalities of the portal, including predetermined PHI authorized for release, messaging capabilities, appointment scheduling capabilities, and the mechanics of transferring of PHI. After determining the functionalities, vendor proposals should be solicited. Once a vendor is selected, an implementation plan in collaboration with the vendor should be developed. Rollout of the portal system should include the following steps: a realistic timeline, defined portal content, testing of access and authentication, and information governance. A timeline helps to ensure goals and objectives are met. Portal content should line up with meaningful use requirements. Implementation testing and ongoing testing are necessary to ensure regulatory compliance. Information governance is necessary to ensure data integrity.

Health Information Exchange

HIE

Health Information Exchange (HIE) refers to the electronic method of accessing and/or sharing patient health information (PHI) among healthcare providers as well as allowing patients to access their own information through secure web-based portals. The capability of electronically accessing and sharing PHI is an efficient means to improve the quality of patient care. Timely sharing of PHI improves decision making at the point of care. It reduces the number of medication errors and eliminates duplicate testing. HIE is a key component of successful healthcare reform. It promotes the interoperability and meaningful used of health information. Through the means of HIE, healthcare costs are reduced.

Types

Health Information Exchange (HIE) refers to the electronic method of accessing and/or sharing patient health information (PHI) among healthcare providers as well as allowing patients to access their own information through secure web-based portals. The 3 types of health information exchange are direct, query-based, and consumer-mediated. Direct exchange occurs between healthcare providers to coordinate care. Examples of direct exchange information that may be shared are laboratory tests results and discharge summaries. Query-based exchange occurs when providers request information, usually for unplanned episodes of care such as an emergency department visit. Consumer-mediated exchange is available for patients to control the use of their PHI among providers (eg, identifying and correcting incorrect health information).

Benefits

Health Information Exchange (HIE) refers to the electronic method of accessing and/or sharing patient health information (PHI) among healthcare providers as well as allowing patients to access their own information through secure web-based portals. The many benefits to electronic health information exchange include:

- Reduction in medication errors because the provider is able to see what drugs have already been prescribed or what dosages have been provided.
- Reduction in medical errors because the provider can access information quickly to obtain knowledge about diagnoses and prognosis.
- Quality of patient care improved as healthcare providers are able to administer more effective care and treatment secondary to the availability of PHI.
- Reduction in paperwork as communication between providers occurs electronically.
- Elimination of duplicate testing because providers are able to know which tests have already been completed.
- Promotes interoperability between electronic health records (EHRs) among healthcare providers.
- Reduction in healthcare costs secondary to time saved pertaining to the completion of paperwork.

ONC

The Office of the National Coordinator for Health Information Technology (ONC) is responsible for leading the movement to promote health information exchange (HIE). HIE is growing in popularity among healthcare providers. As a result, the ONC has established a common set of guiding principles as part of the nationwide strategy to endorse HIE. The guiding principles include:

- Establishment of clear goals for HIE;
- Establishment of measures of success;
- Development of policies and standards;
- Identification of interoperability issues and associated costs; and,
- Inclusion of the patient in the control of his/her health information.

Approach to interoperability enhancement

Despite advances in the adoption of electronic health records (EHRs), challenges remain. There continues to be a lack of standardization, interoperability limitations, and difficulties pertaining to health information exchange (HIE) and access. Hence, the ONC has identified focus areas for improvement. These improvement opportunities emphasize:

- promotion of the use of nationally recognized standards;
- payment methodology reform; and,
- patient awareness of HIE and access.

Nationally recognized standards may be promoted through interoperability protocols such as Fast Healthcare Interoperability Resources (FHIR). The popularity of FHIR is driven by mobile healthcare applications and the cloud, medical device integration, and flexible customizable workflows. The Medicare Access and CHIP Reauthorization Act (MACRA) is instrumental in payment reform. Payment reform examples are the Merit-based Incentive Payment System (MIPS) and the Advanced Alternative Payment Models (APMs). These payment models are linked directly to healthcare treatment quality. Patient awareness of HIE and access will focus on ensuring that all patients know their health information, and HIE will be available to providers and will be exchanged and used among them for the enhancement of their health care.

HL7's approach to interoperability

HL7, or Health Level Seven, along with American Health Information Management Association (AHIMA) subject matter experts, have defined interoperability as "the ability to capture, communicate and exchange data accurately, effectively, securely, and consistently with different information technology systems, software applications, and networks in various settings, and exchange data such that clinical or operational purpose and meaning of the data are preserved and unaltered" (*Journal of AHIMA*, Nov-Dec 2016, p. 55). HL7's approach to interoperability is built on 3 components: semantic, technical, and functional interoperability. Each of these components are further defined as follows:

- Semantic: sharing of content or the ability to correctly interpret information between the sender and receiver;
- Technical: exchange infrastructure; and,
- Functional: rules of information exchange or the ability to correctly share, capture, and use the data according to standardized rules.

Management of HIE process by HIM professionals

HIM professionals involved in the management of the health information exchange (HIE) process should consider several management components. For starters, HIE standards must be developed. The standards should address quality of data content, data algorithms or mapping, and clinical

- 47 -

documentation expectations. Not only should standards be developed, but the data exchange model should be determined. The model should support the entity's or region's health information organization's vision and goals. Determination of what information will be exchanged and what information will not be shared are important components of the HIE process. Of course, this lends to the development of privacy and security policies. HIE management will involve a clear definition of data ownership and stewardship; in other words, data access, use, and control must be consistently monitored. With access to patient information, the opportunity for data to become corrupt is a real possibility. HIM professionals will need to manage a data quality assurance program.

RHIO

A Regional Healthcare Information Organization (RHIO) is a group of healthcare organizations and stakeholders who exchange data electronically. RHIOs are located within the same geographical area. RHIOs must establish a governance structure to include their vision, goals, purpose, and data-sharing needs. The development of an RHIO is an extensive process that may originate in the following manner:

- Development of a strategic plan (which would include the governance structure, vision, goals, etc.).
- Design of detailed functional and operational system requirements. This phase would include determination of data sources, gap analysis studies, determination of reporting requirements, etc.
- Implementation of application build, interface design, network configurations, etc. Training, testing, and data linking evaluations would be a part of the implementation phase.
- Evaluation of its performance against its goals. This can be conducted through analysis of audit trails, monitoring of reports reflecting duplicate records or incorrect information released, and/or analysis of data integration failures.

Information Integrity and Data Quality

Retrieving archived medical information

As patient health information ages and electronic storage space becomes limited, it is necessary for healthcare institutions to archive the information in accordance with federal and state regulatory retention guidance. Once the data are archived, they cannot be changed or deleted prior to their retention guidance, and this principle is known as immutability. The immutability of data ensures the authenticity of the data from a legal perspective. Since large amounts of archived data will need to be maintained for potentially a long period of time, storage space can be of concern; however, technology allows for intelligent compression of the data and this process reduces the amount of storage space. In order to locate archived medical information, effective indexing and searching techniques must be employed. Security of medical information data must be incorporated into the archival process.

Steps to follow during disasters

Inevitably, disasters will occur in the healthcare environment, whether it is a temporary disruption of power or complete destruction of an office. Four levels of disruptions of service constitute the severity of a disaster: limited (eg, power outage), serious (eg, equipment breakdown), major (eg, complete loss of equipment due to flood damage), and catastrophic (eg, complete destruction of an office due to fire). A contingency plan should be in place to recover the loss of data. An important component of the contingency plan would be to routinely back up electronic files. File backups should occur at least daily, and possibly even more frequently (eg, every 8 hours) depending on the volume of data being processed. Backup media should be stored offsite, and backup via cloud services should be considered as well.

Master patient index

The master patient index (MPI) is a data repository of all patients who have ever been admitted or treated at a healthcare organization. The MPI is the source of truth to reference when attempting to locate patient records. The American Hospital Association (AHA) requires that certain patient information be maintained in the MPI (e.g., patient's full name, address, identifying number such as an account number and/or medical record number, and patient's birth date). Sometimes, additional information may be included such as gender, ethnicity, admission/discharge dates, and discharge disposition. Prior to the onset of the electronic health record, the MPI was managed by preparing an index card for every patient, which was maintained in an alphabetical file. The MPI in the electronic world collects the same data as the old manual systems. The electronic MPI is often created by and accessible from electronic health records, and in large healthcare systems, there will likely be an enterprise master patient index (EMPI). An EMPI links together smaller MPIs that are contained within separate systems, such as outpatient clinics, rehab facilities, and hospitals.

Management of patient identification

Accurate and consistent patient identification is an absolute necessity in today's healthcare environment, especially with an emphasis on patient safety. Without proper patient identification, the possibilities of medication administration errors or blood transfusion administration errors can be a reality with unfortunate consequences. A healthcare entity must have an effectively managed master patient index (MPI) or enterprise master patient index (EMPI). Common inconsistencies in MPI or EMPI platforms are duplicates and overlays. Duplicates refer to one patient with multiple medical record numbers or other patient identifiers, and overlays refer to two patient records incorporated into one medical record number. Both can cause serious adverse patient events, and it is imperative that health information management (HIM) departments supervise the MPI/EMPI daily.

Retention requirements

The master patient index (MPI) is a data repository of all patients who have ever been admitted or treated at a healthcare organization. The MPI may be a manual or electronic system. For manual systems, the index cards containing the patient information may be retained in an incorruptible format, such as microfilm or microfiche, and may be kept onsite or offsite. For electronic indices, the patient information should be retained in archived state. The recommended retention period for these indices is at least 10 years, unless state law specifies a different time frame. It is important to remember to always follow the strictest regulation. Retention time frames are influenced by federal and state laws, Medicare, and statute of limitations.

Accurate patient matching at registration

Accuracy of patient identification at the time of registration is an ongoing challenge for healthcare organizations today. Collaboration between centralized and decentralized registration areas is essential to obtaining accurate patient information. A data integrity team of key information professionals should be organized to identify and correct patient identification problems between the various registration areas. Ongoing staff training of key staff must be consistently applied as well. The training should emphasize the long-term effects of poor registration practices, stressing the importance of obtaining viable information, such as previous treatment at the present facility,

- 49 -

nicknames, correct spelling of name, legal name on birth certificate, and even correct punctuation in names. Patient registration clerks should be monitored to ensure that important steps are not overlooked during registration.

Tools to address patient identification

Integration of various tools into the registration process can assist in the validation of patient identity. For example, biometric tools are available to scan palm veins, retinas, and fingerprints. Biometric technology scans vein patterns (whether in the palms or behind the retinas), which are unique patient identifiers. This protects against identity fraud, and enhances the registration process because it minimizes the need to re-enter patient information in subsequent healthcare visits. Registrars can use a valid photo ID or driver's license to validate identity, as well as facial recognition software, and address verification cross-referenced against US Postal Service standards.

Benefits of using biometrics

Biometrics can be defined as a metrics system related to unique human characteristics. The use of biometrics during patient registration processes can reduce, or even potentially eliminate, duplicates as well as improve the accuracy of patient identity matching between multiple healthcare settings and disparate systems. Biometric software has the ability to scan fingerprints, retinas, or veins in the palms. This type of registration process would ensure reliable patient identification. In the present day, few healthcare entities use biometrics during the registration process.

Using data analytics to uncover failed patient merges

Through the use of effective data analytics, it is possible for HIM professionals to identify instances wherein patient information may not have merged into one electronic record. For example, if an information merge from disparate systems fails, patient information is then kept isolated from a consolidated record. This scenario is a risk to the patient's health and safety. A data analytics program can be developed through Excel Pivot tables and/or Access queries to search the database for the unidentified records. For example, newborns are commonly referenced as "Baby Girl" or "Baby Boy" at birth. Their names should be updated to their given name at a future time, but if this process is not carried out, then their information could potentially never be matched with future healthcare occurrences. Data analytics should be used to query for the generic names and their possible matches with legal names through matching patient identifiers, such as social security numbers.

Revenue Management

Revenue Cycle & Reimbursement

Re-sequencing ICD-10-CM codes for optimal reimbursement

When assigning ICD-10-CM codes for an inpatient encounter, there are occasions when it would be appropriate to re-sequence the codes in order to obtain optimal reimbursement. This usually occurs when the ICD-10 Official Coding Guideline for selection of the principal diagnosis is referenced (Section IIC). The Section IIC guideline is used when 2 or more diagnoses equally meet the definition for the principal diagnosis. Of course, the coder must ensure that both diagnoses were determined to be the cause of the admission and both were treated therapeutically or "worked up" with diagnostic procedures. If all of these factors are met, then either diagnosis may be sequenced first. An example of when this guideline could be applied follows: A patient was admitted with exacerbation of chronic obstructive pulmonary disease (COPD) and acute on chronic diastolic heart failure. Both conditions were treated with intravenous meds, oxygen therapy, and respiratory therapy. Since both diagnoses were the reason for the patient's admission and both were treated equally, either one could be selected as the principal diagnosis. Subsequently, the one associated with a higher-weighted DRG should be chosen as the principal diagnosis.

DRG weights

Diagnosis-related groups, or DRGs, as they are better known, are a group of related conditions/diseases that are a component of the inpatient prospective payment system (IPPS). The IPPS is a payment system set forth by the Social Security Act for Medicare Part A recipients that reimburses healthcare entities for their operating expenses associated with the provision of acute care inpatient stays. Each DRG has its own unique weight based on the average amount of resources used to treat patients who fall into that category. Those conditions that are costly will be categorized in a higher-weighted DRG. To calculate a DRG reimbursement rate, a standardized amount for labor and non-labor components, wage index factor, cost of living adjustment, and earnings by occupational category are all calculated into the reimbursement rate.

Payment models

Obtaining reimbursement for healthcare services is a complex process. It is imperative that the coding department and the financial services' (or revenue cycle) department communicate efficiently and effectively in order to obtain maximum reimbursement. There are several different payment models in the healthcare arena currently. A well-known payment model is the traditional fee-for-service model. This model requires payers to reimburse each service performed. Value-based delivery care is making changes in reimbursement methodologies. This model will move away from the traditional fee-for-service model. Accountable care organizations (ACOs) are a type of value-based delivery care, wherein a large health system shares its savings by managing patients' health for less money. Incentivized payment models reward physicians for meeting certain quality and efficiency goals. Payment bundling and payment per case (eg, DRG) continue to be popular methods of reimbursement.

Updating a charge ticket for a hospital

In order to prevent payer denials, a hospital should update departmental charge tickets annually (at a minimum) or as significant coding/charging changes occur. The same changes should be coordinated with the hospital chargemaster. By proactively making the necessary changes to a charge ticket and the chargemaster, denials on the back end are reduced or avoided. It is best to review ICD-10 and CPT codes as they are updated annually to ensure the departmental tickets and chargemaster include the updates. Code descriptions should be assessed to ensure that the terminology is correct and not misleading to a health professional who might select the wrong code/charge based on an incorrect title.

Chargemaster

Purpose

A hospital has a database that contains all charges for services rendered. This database is known as the chargemaster or charge description master (CDM). The CDM is the core of a hospital's revenue cycle. Each hospital department is responsible for entering the type of service or supply provided to a patient. Each procedure, supply, or service has its own unique item number. For each charge, a CPT/HCPCS code and revenue code as well as other financial elements are assigned. The functions of the CDM are to not only assign charges, but also to produce itemized statements, produce a valid claim, monitor costs, and generate financial reporting.

Elements

A hospital's chargemaster is composed of certain key elements. The typical data elements are the following:

- Charge description: Each charge has a title that describes the charge whether it is a supply, a medication, a procedure, etc.
- CPT/HCPCS code and modifiers: A CPT or HCPCS code may be assigned to a specific procedure or supply, and applicable modifiers may be built in to the charge as well. Of note, not all charges will have a corresponding CPT/HCPCS code or modifier.
- Revenue code: This is a 3-digit number that represents the location of the patient when the service was rendered or the type of service the patient received.
- Charge dollar amount: This is the cost associated with the service or supply provided.
- Charge code: This is the unique number assigned to each item listed in the chargemaster. It is also known as the CDM number.
- Charge status: This represents whether or not the charge has been allocated to the patient's account and its payment or denial status.

DNFB

DNFB is the abbreviation for "discharged, not final billed." It is a familiar term used in medical coding practices, and refers to those accounts wherein the patient has been discharged from the hospital, but the account has not been final billed yet. DNFB status is applicable to those accounts that fall within usually a 4- to 5-day billing hold period after discharge and are still in need of code assignments. DNFB is important because it is a vital part of the revenue cycle, affecting the bottom line. It significantly impacts account receivable (A/R) days. The DNFB is calculated by dividing the gross revenue for the month by the days in the month, which provides the average daily gross revenue. For example, $120 million/30 days = $4 million daily. The dollar amount of accounts discharged but not billed is then divided by the average daily gross revenue monthly amount. For example, $28 million/$4 million = 7 days. A range pertaining to an acceptable number of days (eg, 6.2 to 7 days = excellent; 7.1 to 8.2 days = caution; >8.3 days = needs immediate attention/action).

Revenue cycle management

Revenue cycle management in healthcare is a 3-part process. It involves management of the healthcare institution's claims processing, payment processing, and revenue generation. The revenue cycle begins at the point of determining patient eligibility, collecting the patient's copay and/or deductible, correct coding of claims, correct charging of services, tracking claims between the provider and the payer, collecting payments, and claims denial management. Two other factors impact revenue for a healthcare entity: provider/physician productivity and patient volume (admissions/ discharges/ transfers).

Claim denials

Insurance claim denials are an expected occurrence in healthcare revenue cycle management. Common claim denials and an explanation are as follows:

Type of Denial	Explanation
Technical	Denials may occur because of a problem with claims processing
Logic-based	Denials may occur when an ICD-10-CM or CPT code does not match a PCS code.
Unspecified codes	ICD-10 coding allows for more code specificity, and unspecified codes raise red flags with payers.
Medical necessity	Denials may occur if medical necessity conditions are not met according to NCDs and LCDs.
Insurance eligibility	Denials may occur when the provider bills the wrong insurance payer.
Modifiers	Denials are likely to occur with modifier -25 or -59 as these two modifiers are commonly misused.

Tools for tracking denials

Part of the revenue cycle management process is to track insurance payer denials and trend the reasons for the denials so that future denials can be prevented. Healthcare entities should use certain tools for the purpose of tracking denials. A claim denial spreadsheet can be used to track the reasons for denials, follow-up status, identify areas responsible for denials, and show impact on income. Dashboards are useful to display department-specific data compared against benchmarks. Trending of data can be incorporated into the dashboards as well. Denial tracking by payer is another useful tool. One can identify and quantify such data for trending purposes.

Adjudication

Adjudication in the revenue cycle management world is a process in which submitted claims are evaluated by the payer for validity and determination of whether payment will be rendered or not. It is during the adjudication process that a claim will be accepted, denied, or rejected. Accepted means that the payer has decided the claim is valid, but the payer may not reimburse the claim in full. They are required to process the claim according to the subscriber's plan (e.g., an 80/20 plan). A denied claim, of course, means the payer has found reason to refuse payment for the services rendered (e.g., failure to meet medical necessity). A rejected claim identified during the adjudication process means that the payer has identified a claim error. A rejected claim may be resubmitted by the provider for reconsideration.

Medicare appeals process for claim denials

When a healthcare provider disagrees with Medicare's payment decision (Part A), an appeal may be pursued. The appeal process can be lengthy as there are 5 levels of appeal. Level 1 involves a redetermination process by the company who processes claims for Medicare. Level 2 involves reconsideration by a qualified independent contractor (QIC). Level 3 would be pursued if the claim needs to be presented to an administrative law judge (ALJ). If not successful at that level, the claim can be reviewed by the Medicare Appeals Council (Level 4). A final attempt for appeal can be a judicial review in a federal district court. Each level has certain requirements to follow, and time frames can be rather long (eg, 180 days).

Generating clean claims

For a healthcare entity to have a 100% clean claim rate would be nothing short of a miracle. The reality is there are many challenges with submitting clean claims; however, there are strategies to follow that can reduce the number of "dirty" claims and thus reduce the number of denials. One key strategy would be for a healthcare provider to scrub claims before submitting them to the clearinghouse and/or the insurance payer. Through the process of scrubbing claims, errors are identified and routed to the appropriate personnel within the healthcare entity, who can correct the errors before dropping the claim. In order for this process to be effective, it is beneficial for the healthcare provider to be familiar with all payer edits. Careful analysis of the reasons why claims are rejected by edits is beneficial to understand as well. This ties into another strategy of staying abreast of healthcare revenue trends as well as being vigilant in the ever-changing world of governmental regulations.

Preventing denials through proper training and up-to-date resources

One of the critical steps a healthcare provider can conduct is to ensure that all revenue cycle resources are current. This requires updating of resources at least annually, and for some resources (eg, chargemaster), updating may be more frequent. Obviously, the current version of ICD-10 and CPT codes must be referenced. With the transition to ICD-10 from ICD-9 on October 1, 2015, all healthcare providers should be up-to-date with coding changes. However, it is important to note that beginning October 1, 2016, even more ICD-10 code changes are forthcoming for the fiscal year 2017. Encounter forms or charge slips should be updated when services change or charging errors are identified. The current versions of national coverage determinations (NCDs) and local coverage determinations (LCDs) should be referenced, as well as the current edits. Utilization of the current versions of any revenue-based resource will help to reduce denials.

Regulatory

Hospital accreditation

Hospital accreditation is a peer assessment process conducted by an external agency whose primary purpose is to evaluate healthcare performance against established standards and then recommend steps to improve delivery of healthcare. The Joint Commission is the nation's top accreditor for hospitals. The Joint Commission will award a gold seal of approval, which is internationally recognized, when a hospital meets the evidence-based standards pertaining to quality of care and patient safety. All types of hospitals (e.g., government-owned, long-term rehab, psychiatric) and treatment provided by facilities (e.g., home health, ambulatory care) after hospitalization can achieve accreditation. In addition to accreditation services, Joint Commission promotes performance improvement to help the healthcare organization succeed even after the accreditation process is over. Additional certifications may be granted in addition to the Joint Commission accreditation status, such as disease-specific care certifications, patient blood management, medication compounding, etc.

Becoming accredited by Joint Commission

Before the initial Joint Commission survey is conducted, the healthcare organization should complete the following steps, at a minimum:

- Ensure the state licensure requirements have been met.
- Ensure the CMS 855A application has been verified.
- Ensure that patient census requirements are met in order to provide an ample supply of records to The Joint Commission surveyors.
- Request a free trial edition of the The Joint Commission standards.
- Request an Accreditation Guide.
- Apply for Accreditation Survey and pay the nonrefundable fee.

Before the survey has ended, The Joint Commission surveyors will schedule an exit conference to review a preliminary summary of findings. The preliminary report may be further reviewed by The Joint Commission's Central Office. Once the review is finalized, a final summary will be posted on the The Joint Commission's extranet site. Post-survey requests for additional information may be submitted by The Joint Commission with time limits set for either 45 or 60 days. These are known as Evidence of Standards Compliance (ESC) requests. Once these are submitted by the healthcare organization, the accreditation decision will be rendered.

Healthcare compliance audit

Multiple types of healthcare compliance audits are being conducted in the present age. To understand the purpose of a compliance audit, it is important to understand the different types of audits. Hospitals should be prepared in the following areas (at a minimum) where audits are likely to occur: HIPAA, meaningful use, provider-based status, outlier payments, Medicare's Two-Midnight Rule, Inpatient Claims for Mechanical Ventilation, Ambulatory Surgery Centers Payment System, Anesthesia Services, Outpatient Rehab Services, Immunosuppressive Drug Claims, Hospice and Home Health Services, etc. The list of potential audits by external agencies is extensive. The Office of Inspector General (OIG) publishes a Work Plan for each fiscal year, and this plan is an excellent indicator of where hospitals, skilled nursing facilities, pharmacies, clinics, etc., should focus their attention for internal auditing. The purpose behind each of these external auditors essentially is to identify fraud, waste, and abuse. They are looking for opportunities to improve healthcare efficiency, and in many cases this includes holding accountable those who violate federal healthcare laws.

Governmental audits

Federal auditors have the authority to review Medicare and Medicaid claims submitted by providers. Federal government audit entities are Medicare Recovery Audit Contractor (RAC), Office of Inspector General (OIG), Zone Program Integrity Contractor (ZPIC), and Department of Justice (DOJ). Depending on the entity involved, the auditor will have different scopes of work, and the number of accounts reviewed, timeline of the audit, and appeals process will vary among the auditors. The RAC's goal is to reduce Medicare improper payments. The focus of the OIG, DOJ, and ZPICs is on fraud and abuse. It is imperative that healthcare organizations be prepared for governmental audits.

External audits that may be requested of a hospital

Hospitals experience audits from external agencies on a regular basis. The external auditors may be representatives of various federal agencies (e.g., Office of Inspector General, Department of Justice, Medicare Administrative Contractors). They may represent commercial insurers (e.g., Blue Cross/Blue Shield). The types of audits requested may pertain to charges (e.g., pharmaceutical, supplies), coding, medical necessity, fraud, etc. Complete and detailed documentation is key to proving to the external auditor that a submitted claim is valid and meets regulatory compliance.

EMTALA audit

Congress enacted the Emergency Medical Treatment and Labor Act (EMTALA) in 1986 to ensure that all people would have access to emergency services regardless of the individual's ability to pay. This Act mandates hospitals to provide stabilizing treatment for a patient with an emergency medical condition, and if unable to stabilize the patient, the hospital is required to transfer the patient to a facility where stabilization can occur. EMTALA is enforced by CMS as well as the Office of Inspector General (OIG), and either entity may conduct an audit. To prepare for an EMTALA audit, hospitals should review their EMTALA and transfer policies and procedures (P&Ps), medical staff bylaws, physician on-call lists, emergency workflows, emergency department transfer form, and emergency department signage. P&Ps should be up-to-date with EMTALA guidance. Medical staff bylaws should indicate who is allowed to perform the medical screening exam. The emergency workflow should be EMTALA compliant, and signage should be easy to understand and follow from the patient's perspective. The transfer forms must be completed in their entirety, and on-call lists must correspond with documentation in the medical record.

Preparing for external audits

Hospitals experience audits from external agencies on a regular basis. The external auditors may be representatives of various federal agencies (e.g., Office of Inspector General, Department of Justice, Medicare Administrative Contractors). They may represent commercial insurers (e.g., Blue Cross/Blue Shield). The types of audits requested may pertain to charges (e.g., pharmaceutical, supplies), coding, medical necessity, fraud, contracts, policies, etc. Preparation should include the development and implementation of policies and procedures, organizational education regarding each department's responsibility during an audit, identification of individuals internally who should be involved in the audits, and determination of appeals processes.

Pre-bill and retrospective coding audits

A pre-bill coding audit is an audit that is conducted before the initial claim is ever submitted to the payer. The benefit to conducting a pre-bill audit is that errors are identified and corrected proactively, which prevents payment denials and/or payment take-backs by the payer. A pre-bill audit provides an opportunity for the auditor to identify any "red flags," which alert governmental payers of potential errors through their data analysis software. Pre-bill audits result in high reimbursement for providers because repetitive paybacks are reduced or eliminated. On the contrary, a retrospective coding audit is performed after the initial claim has been submitted to the payer, and if errors are identified during the audit, a subsequent bill with corrected errors is submitted. This results in extra work effort for the billing department and can raise red flags with payers.

Effective coding audit program

Effective coding compliance audit programs should incorporate the following elements, at a minimum: high-risk cases (e.g., excisional debridement, mechanical ventilation), cases with a DRG shift between ICD-9 and ICD-10 coding conventions, surgical procedure cases that require several codes for accurate reporting (e.g., spinal fusion with diskectomy), hospital-acquired conditions (HACs), unspecified codes, and resource intensive DRGs. Challenges facing effective coding compliance audit programs may be: insufficient documentation, insufficient physician queries, difficulties in understanding ICD-10-PCS procedural coding logic, difficulties in understanding how to code multiple complex procedures, misunderstanding of root operation definitions and applications, and failure to code to the highest level of specificity. Despite the challenges, effective coding audit programs are achievable and many opportunities exist going forward to educate and mentor coding professionals to become subject matter experts.

Medical chart audit

The objective and goals of chart audits may be related to research, compliance, financial, or clinical reasons. Wherever issues are discovered to be noncompliant with federal or state regulations or healthcare policies and procedures, an audit may be conducted. The primary purpose is to determine the extent of noncompliance, how the issues should be corrected, and how to prevent the issues from occurring again. A beneficial use of a medical chart audit is to measure the quality of care and improve upon it. Examples of audit types for medical chart audits include: preventive care (such as the percentage of women in a certain age range who have a mammogram annually) and chronic disease management (such as the percentage of patients with hypertension whose medication was adjusted multiple times during the year). The steps involved in conducting a medical chart audit should be:

- Select an audit focus that is not too broad or too narrow and one that is a high risk to the healthcare entity.
- Define the audit criteria and how to measure the information against the criteria.
- Identify the patient population.
- Determine the sample size (results need to be statistically valid, so the sample size is critical).
- Determine audit tools to utilize (e.g., tools that can calculate rates, percentages, or other statistical measurements).
- Collect data.
- Summarize, analyze, and apply results for comparison against benchmarks.

Continuous monitoring process

Continuous monitoring can be defined as an automated means to assess risk on a frequent basis. Continuous monitoring may assess a high-risk area on a quarterly basis, and once improvement is noted or the risk is lowered, then continuous monitoring will cease. Data analysis tools are essential to the process of continuous monitoring because these tools are instrumental in identifying data exceptions or anomalies and/or analyzing patterns. The identified exceptions that fail to meet criteria or standards are subsequently audited for potential noncompliance. To implement a continuous monitoring program, a healthcare entity should identify and establish priority high-risk areas, identify continuous auditing rules, determine the frequency of the audits, determine the parameters, determine follow-up procedures, and determine result communication procedures.

Internal auditor qualifications

The International Standards for the Professional Practice of Internal Auditing identifies several qualifications for internal auditors. These standards are applicable for internal auditors as well as the overall audit activity within an organization. The purpose of the standards is to provide a framework of guidance for internal auditors so that auditing consistency and compliance is promoted within the organization. Key qualifications or expectations include the following:

- Internal auditors must be objective in performing their work in order to prevent bias.
- Internal auditors must avoid conflicts of interest.
- Audits must be performed with proficiency and due professional care.
- Internal auditors must stay current with their knowledge and skills through continuing educational opportunities.
- Internal auditors must not audit operations for which they were previously responsible.

Management of internal audit activities

The chief compliance officer (CCO) or chief audit executive (CAE) must effectively manage the internal audit program of a healthcare organization. Effective management of the program will conform to the International Standards for the Professional Practice of Internal Auditing. Effective management of the program will be evident through compliance with the organization's Code of Ethics. As part of the management process, the CCO or CAE must develop an audit plan based on a risk-based approach, meaning that all organizational risks must be identified and then scored in order to determine those areas of highest risk. Senior management throughout the organization provides insight into perceived risks. Based on the risk analysis, an audit plan is developed and subsequently approved by the board of directors. The approved audit plan can be amended throughout the fiscal year depending on new risks, new or revised operations, changes in controls, etc.

Steps of an internal healthcare compliance audit

When preparing for an audit, internal auditors must develop an audit framework that will address the audit's scope, objectives, timing, and risks. The process should begin by holding an entrance conference with management of the audited area to identify risks relevant to the activity under review. Resources and pertinent criteria must be identified and referenced during the audit process. Types of resources and criteria may be federal and/or state regulations, organizational policies and procedures, and leading practices (e.g., professional guidance, benchmarks). The scope should include acknowledgement of relevant electronic systems, records (whether paper or electronic based), staff, and property. The objectives should note all parameters such as population size and time frame. Analysis and evaluation of documentation and data will be instrumental for the auditor to draw conclusions and subsequently communicate the findings to administration. The auditor must keep detailed and extensive documentation to support the audit findings.

Coding

Encoder

An encoder is an electronic tool that receives diagnostic or procedural data manually entered by a coder, which then converts the data into a numerical code. An encoder is a logic-driven tool that prompts the coder through several choices/options until the appropriate code is achieved. This tool promotes consistency and accuracy because it potentially prevents the coder from missing a key piece of information. In many computer-assisted coding (CAC) programs, the encoder is an integral part. The encoder serves the same purpose in CAC as it does in a stand-alone encoder—logically guide the coder to the appropriate code selection based on the providers' documentation. Whether a coder uses a stand-alone encoder, a CAC encoder, or codes with an ICD-10 book only, the critical skill for the coder is to accurately and thoroughly search the health information for the diagnoses and procedures that affect the hospital stay.

CAC

Computer-assisted coding (CAC) software is a helpful aid to coders in that it analyzes electronic health information for specific medical terms and phrases that correlate to numerical codes. CAC software uses natural language processing (NLP) to identify the terminology. CAC offers many benefits to a coder, such as efficiency in coding, increased production, decrease in average coding turnaround time, consistency in following coding guidelines, and decreased coding error rates. Even though coding errors rates may decrease, it is still imperative for a coder to double-check the CAC-assigned codes because CAC is capable of selecting incorrect terminology. For example, CAC may select cancer as a diagnosis to code, but in reality, the appropriate code should reflect *history of cancer*.

NLP processing

Natural Language Processing (NLP) is an integral and important part of computer-assisted coding (CAC). NLP technology has the capability to process text as well as data fields containing text into suggested ICD-10 codes. NLP technologies differ in how they decipher narrative texts, how they recognize coding-related data, and how they integrate data between systems. An efficient CAC system will be one that correctly suggests accurate codes based on coding and/or regulatory guidelines, and through the CAC's accuracy, the coder's job is more easily accomplished. In other words, if a CAC-recommended code has supporting documentation and is an accurate recommendation, the coder can review the suggested code and documentation more quickly, thus increasing production. The best CAC system will operate with an NLP with excellent encoder functionality so that the coder does not have to access various systems of an encoder, coding references, EHR, etc.

Auditing code assignments

Healthcare entities should never assume that computer-assisted coding (CAC) systems are 100% accurate. It is imperative to implement a coding compliance program in which auditors review accounts on a daily basis. The volume of coded charts will far outweigh the number of auditors available to review. Appropriate data analysis and filtering methods should be implemented to identify high-risk accounts. Once automated auditing tools identify the high-risk accounts, a systematic approach of auditing for compliant coding practices should occur. Any coding discrepancies should be conveyed to the coder for corrections and/or further discussion. After recommended corrections are made, rebills of corrected claims to the appropriate payer should occur.

Potential problems with CAC-assigned codes

Computer-assisted coding (CAC) software does not diminish the role of a coder. Rather, the value of having the coder's knowledge and skills applied to the CAC process enhances the overall coding accuracy. In other words, coders will not be replaced by a machine because problems do exist with CAC. One potential problem with CAC-assigned codes pertains to the software's inability to logically decipher complicated cases, and therefore it is necessary for a coder to comprehend the coding rules correctly and assign the appropriate code(s). Another known CAC-related problem is with the software's inability to decipher current illnesses versus historical illnesses as well as illnesses related to family diseases versus personal history.

Fraud Surveillance

Medical identity theft

Medical identity theft is on the rise. The impact on patients can be devastating as the breach may result in criminals maximizing health benefits of the victim's insurance plan, or the criminal may be successful in obtaining prescription drugs. For example, thieves may hold health information ransom, demanding large sums of money to return the health information to the patient or healthcare entity. Health information management (HIM) professionals should be involved in mitigating the risks associated with medical identity theft. HIM professionals can build awareness that medical identity is a patient safety issue. They can provide staff education on how to identify fraudulent activity. They can work with Information Technology (IT) in mitigating phishing scams and initiating valid pass code applications. HIM professionals can assist in identifying fraudulent activity through data analysis and the performance of proactive audits.

Cybersecurity plan

While Information Technology (IT) departments are the key individuals responsible for the security of health information, Health Information Management (HIM) professionals should be involved since they are knowledgeable of information workflows. Healthcare entities are wise to use their IT staff as well as HIM staff to proactively implement cybersecurity plans for the purpose of preventing cybercriminal activities. A cybersecurity plan should include a risk assessment of all software applications used by the healthcare entity. The risk assessment should look for protection gaps, and the identified vulnerable systems should be patched to close the weakness. Encryption is another vital method that should be used in the fight against cyber theft. All workstations and portable mediums should be encrypted. Encryption is effective in that it scrambles the data so that it cannot be deciphered by people or electronic systems.

Steps CMS is taking regarding medical identity theft

The Centers for Medicare and Medicaid Services (CMS) is aware of medical identity theft and the various techniques thieves are using to steal information. CMS is especially concerned with one piece of information thieves target, which is social security numbers. An effective deterrent being actively pursued is the removal of the social security number from the Medicare/Medicaid card. The new Medicare Access and CHIP Reauthorization Act (MACRA) requires the US Department of Health and Human Services (HHS) to collaborate with the Commissioner of Social Security to ensure that social security numbers are not included on the card. This is known as the Social Security Number Removal Initiative (SSNRI). By 2018, the card will include a randomly assigned Medicare Beneficiary Identifier (MBI) instead of a social security number. The new MBI must be used in all healthcare interactions. This initiative will minimize the risk of identity theft for Medicare/Medicaid beneficiaries. In consideration of this initiative, HIM professionals should be involved in healthcare policy revisions regarding whether or not social security numbers should even be collected going forward. If it is determined the social security number is still needed, then HIM professionals should assist with determining how it will be stored and who will have access to it.

Medical identity theft response program

When a medical identity incident occurs, the healthcare entity must promptly respond. As part of the program requirements, patients affected by identity theft must be notified of the incident. The privacy officer, health information management, financial accounting, and involved physicians should be notified. A faux medical record should be created that includes the thief's information. The affected patient and possibly involved physicians need to be involved in this process to identify what information is accurate and what information is false (fabricated by the thief). Both patient records need to be flagged indefinitely in order to alert all healthcare providers of the medical identity incident. A final step in the program should be that the healthcare entity offers the victim free credit and/or medical identity monitoring services. This service should be provided for a minimum of 3 years.

Investigative methods

When notification from a consumer reporting agency of a medical identity theft incident has occurred, a medical theft response team should act promptly. The Master Patient Index (MPI) should be referenced for accuracy of social security numbers, drivers' license numbers, US passports, legal permanent resident cards, telephone numbers, addresses, etc., aiming to identify discrepancies between the new information and information already on file. Patient signatures on file can be compared to signatures on new documents, looking specifically for signs of forgery. Discrepancies in the spelling of the patient's name, birth date, and/or clinical information (such as height or weight) can be clues of a possible identity theft, as well as invalid addresses and phone numbers. Naturally, if a new patient submits information during registration that is confirmed as belonging to a deceased individual, there should be immediate concerns of attempted identity theft.

Clinical Documentation Improvement

Process when conflicting documentation exists

Patients who are admitted to an inpatient status in the hospital may be assessed by multiple physicians. Inevitably, the documentation of the various physicians will conflict. For example, the attending physician may document acute renal "failure," but the nephrology consultant documents acute renal "disease." Since failure and disease in this particular case equate to different codes, the coder will need clarification, and that clarification is best achieved through the initiation of a query. The query would need to reveal the conflicting information and ask for the final decision as to which diagnosis is correct. Other clinical indicators should be a part of the query in order to demonstrate to the physician why the information is conflicting. For example, in this acute renal failure versus disease scenario, the coder may choose to include the clinical indicators pertaining to a rise in the BUN/creatinine as well as the urine output amounts.

Physician query

Initiation of a physician query is appropriate when documentation within the medical record fails to provide the necessary information needed by the coder to make an informed decision about a code assignment. Issues such as legibility, completeness, clarity, or consistency may prompt the initiation of a query. The query may be done either concurrently by a clinical documentation improvement (CDI) specialist or retrospectively by a coder. Physician queries must be phrased in such a way that it does not appear that the CDI specialist or coder is leading the physician to a certain diagnosis. Physician queries must provide clinical indicators from the existing documentation that explains the CDI specialist's or coder's reasoning to the queried physician.

Intent

A physician query is a tool of communication between CDI specialists/coders and physicians to clarify incomplete, ambiguous, or conflicting documentation in the medical record. The intention of the communication tool is to facilitate completeness, accuracy, consistency, and timely documentation for coding and reporting practices. Queries are an essential tool and provide additional clarification that allows coding and reporting to the highest level of specificity. It is best for the physician's query to be maintained as a permanent part of the medical record since it is considered to be supporting documentation for assigned codes.

Required components

A physician query should include certain components in order to be a valid and/or compliant query. These components should be:

- Name of the contact individual submitting the query
- Patient's date of service (DOS)
- Patient's name
- Medical Record Number
- Account Number
- Date of the query
- Name of the MD being queried
- Clinical indicators pertinent to the condition/diagnosis/procedure in question
- Statement of the issue in the form of a question

Examples of when queries may be issued are:

- Determine if a diagnosis was present on admission (POA).
- Clarify what specific organism was the cause and effect of an infectious disease.
- Clarify the severity of asthma.
- Clarify the particular stage of chronic kidney disease (CKD).
- Clarify if a diagnosis was ruled in or ruled out.
- Determine which diagnosis or procedure is applicable when conflicting information exists.
- Clarify whether or not pneumonia was caused by aspiration.

Clinical indicators

Compliant coding is dependent on the accuracy and completeness of documentation. Healthcare documentation is not sufficient to support code assignments, and in those cases, physician queries are necessary. Queries must contain certain elements, and clinical indicators are one of the elements. Clinical indicators refer to clinical clues, such as elevated temperature, abnormal vital signs, or elevated white blood count levels, which could indicate or support certain diagnoses. For example, if a provider fails to document the diagnosis of sepsis, but there are clinical indicators that point to its diagnosis, a query might be warranted. The coder or clinical documentation improvement (CDI) specialist might include the following clinical indicators in the query: temperature 103°, WBC 18,500, blood pressure 70/40 (hypotension). These 3 clinical clues might indicate the diagnosis of sepsis, and the physician would consider these indicators to make a decision.

Leading query

A leading query can be defined as one that is not supported by the clinical elements contained within the medical record, or it can be defined as a query that directs a healthcare provider to a specific diagnosis or procedure. Leading a provider to a specific diagnosis or procedure is an unbalanced approach because it appears to prompt the provider to make only one decision. A coder or clinical documentation improvement (CDI) specialist should never suggest only one diagnostic or procedural option because coders/CDI specialists are not credentialed healthcare providers.

Leading provider/physician queries are not acceptable in health care. Following are examples of inappropriate leading queries:

- A query that provides the physician with options that only lead to additional reimbursement.
- A query that does not contain all the required clinical indicators to paint the full clinical picture of the patient's condition.
- A query wherein the statements are directive in nature, such as indicating what the provider should document, rather than querying the provider for his/her professional determination of the clinical facts.
- A query that leads the provider to one desired outcome.
- A query that omits reasonable clinically supported options.
- A query that omits an option that no additional documentation or clarification may be provided.

Standardized physician query forms

The use of standardized physician query forms by coders and/or clinical documentation improvement (CDI) specialists is an efficient way to obtain compliant queries. Standardized queries should be created based on disease processes or circumstances that are likely to require a query (e.g., sepsis, acuity of respiratory failure, specificity of renal failure, whether a diagnosis was ruled in or ruled out). Through the utilization of standardized forms with specified clinical indicators, 3 objectives should be accomplished: 1) overall documentation improvement should be noted, 2) potential coding errors due to poor documentation practices should be avoided, and 3) potential compliance issues related to leading queries should be mitigated.

Query formatting options

There are several ways to generate a query: compliant query forms allow for open-ended questions, multiple choice query formats, and/or limited yes/no query formats. An example of open-ended query might appear in this format: "Based on your clinical judgment, please provide a diagnosis that represents the following clinical indicators: temperature 102°, cellulitis around ankle with open wound, white blood cell count 15,000." An example of a multiple-choice query might appear in this format: "Per the Discharge Summary, the patient has congestive heart failure (CHF). Can the CHF be further specified as: 1) acute systolic CHF, 2) acute on chronic systolic CHF, 3) acute diastolic CHF, 4) acute on chronic diastolic CHF, or 5) undetermined?" An example of a yes/no query might appear in this format: "Was the sepsis documented in the Discharge Summary present on admission? Yes, No, clinically unable to determine."

Promoting clinical documentation improvement opportunities with physicians

Physicians are sometimes resistant when it comes to improving their documentation, primarily because of the belief that it entails more work for them to complete. However, there are effective ways to promote clinical documentation improvement among physicians. Examples are:

- Communicate that good clinical documentation is instrumental in supporting quality initiatives and improved patient outcomes.
- Communicate that good clinical documentation affects quality scores related to physician contracts and reimbursement.
- Provide education that explains reimbursement concepts and how clinical documentation impacts the reimbursement methodology.
- Provide meaningful feedback and/or data to all physicians, such as common DRGs, common complications/comorbidities, or risk of mortality scores.
- Provide education pertaining to the effect of documentation problems on medical necessity.

Show examples of claim denials based on poor documentation and how better documentation would have prevented the denial.

Importance of physician query policies

Physician queries are an integral part of clinical documentation improvement (CDI) programs in healthcare institutions today. In order to standardize methods for physician query processes, query policies are recommended. Effective policies should establish query guidelines pertaining to the 4 "Ws" – who (eg, which physician is responsible for providing clarity), what (eg, which diagnosis or procedure is unclear), when (eg, when is a query needed), and why (eg, is documentation unclear or conflicting?). Policies should also address any compliance-related issues (eg, avoidance of leading a physician to the selection of a desired diagnosis). Query policies should explain appropriate means of following up on unanswered queries (eg, time frames, acceptable number of queries to issue).

Clinical documentation improvement

Clinical documentation improvement (CDI) is the process of reviewing health information for conflicting or incomplete provider documentation that fails to support the assignment of diagnostic or procedural codes. The CDI process is critically important because the health record is the primary tool used between clinicians to communicate and ensure continuity of the patient's care. Documentation should always capture the complete and accurate picture of the patient's health status and treatment, and the CDI process ensures the completeness and accuracy. CDI requires buy-in by the provider in order for it to be successful. One of the best ways to "train" each provider or to gain his/her buy-in is to demonstrate to him/her that CDI helps the provider to meet quality measures.

Leadership

Leadership Roles

Implementing a mentoring plan for new coders

With the advent of ICD-10 in October 2015, new coding challenges surfaced. Many seasoned or experienced coders retired, and new coder interest was insufficient. Many healthcare entities have been forced to develop training plans for new coders. These training plans may include a mentorship. An ideal mentorship program would be structured in the following manner: Assign a mentor (an experienced coding professional) to 2 new coders. The mentor will then review 100% of all coded accounts by the new coders prior to billing. The mentor will provide educational feedback to the new coders for each account. The educational feedback should always reference applicable medical information and/or Coding Clinic references. Time should be allotted for the new coders to review the feedback, hold discussions, and review multiple training resources. A key component of this training plan is open communication, especially if mentors and coders work in remote environments.

Great leader skills

Job opportunities in the health information field are abundant and require technical and leadership skills. The following skills are critical to a successful HIM career:

- Confidence - HIM professionals should exert themselves and be noticed by other professionals as possessing an inner strength.
- Drive for Success - HIM professionals should establish goals and take all necessary steps to achieve the goals.
- Innovation - HIM professionals should embrace change and be constantly thinking of new ways to move forward.
- Flexibility - HIM professionals should accept change and be adaptable.
- Integrity - Integrity cultivates trust, and trust by peers and/or subordinates is key to success.
- Collaboration - HIM professionals should be able to build relationships as well as build and develop successful teams.
- Communication - HIM professionals must be able to effectively communicate in verbal and written form, as well as through listening skills.
- Knowledge - HIM professionals should attain knowledge in multiple areas and be lifelong learners.

Building a successful team

Building a team to a level of success will hinge on how well the leader enables each team member to reach his/her best potential and goals. Through team approaches, healthcare entities can experience increased production, customer satisfaction, cost savings, and goal achievements. Leaders should build teams by establishing goals and objectives, by defining responsibilities for each team member, and by recognizing each member's unique contribution to the team. The following steps should be considered when developing teams: Lay out the problem or issue for collaboration. Determine the key stakeholders who need to be included on the team. Establish goals and objectives. Provide direction and then do not micromanage the process; let the team conduct the work. Provide necessary resources to complete tasks. Assess the team's results, provide further direction if needed, and ultimately reward success when goals and objectives are accomplished.

Organization and facilitation of meetings

As a health information management (HIM) professional, organization and facilitation of meetings is a common and frequent responsibility. The meetings may be routine monthly or quarterly staff meetings, administrative meetings, or meetings with clinical professionals (e.g., physicians, nursing, radiology). Organizing and facilitating routine staff meetings tend to follow a prescribed methodology of addressing staff accomplishments, upcoming events, discussions pertaining to identified problems, educational sessions, organization-wide announcements, open discussions, etc. Agendas should be developed and distributed prior to the meeting date for guidance and timeliness purposes. For the more impromptu meetings or non-routine meetings, it is always best to inform the attendees (ahead of the meeting time) of the objectives as well as who will be responsible for speaking to each agenda item. This will help promote the best use of time during the meeting. When facilitating or leading the meeting (regardless of the meeting type), it is essential to be prepared. Know in advance the topics to be discussed and have available any reference materials to review. Think through the agenda items beforehand and develop any pertinent questions that may need to be addressed so that key information will not be overlooked.

Managing virtual meetings

Virtual meetings are a commonplace occurrence in healthcare organizations. Effective management of a virtual meeting requires practice and development of key skills. These skills may include any of the following: Before the meeting, create and distribute an agenda, review the agenda with another individual who can cover the meeting in case you are unexpectedly absent, and practice with the virtual technology. Navigation of the virtual software should be an easy process, so practicing ahead of time will build confidence. When the meeting begins, ask who is in attendance with each "beep" that is heard, and then consider introducing each member and their role in the meeting so everyone will be clear as to their part (if the meeting attendance is large, introductions may be eliminated). Begin the meeting on time in respect of everyone's time, and do not restart with every late comer. Keep the meeting moving along by staying focused and eliminating distractions. Allow time for attendees' input and discussion, and recap the important takeaways of the meeting and who is responsible for follow-up or action steps. After the meeting has concluded, distribute brief minutes/notes, and if the meeting was recorded, distribute an emailed link to the webinar online.

Opportunities to volunteer for AHIMA

The American Health Information Management Association is a professional organization for HIM professionals. As with any professional organization, there are many opportunities to volunteer. In order to identify volunteer opportunities, contact the state associational leadership team and ask about opportunities as well as offer expertise. One type of opportunity may be to serve in a regional or local office (e.g., treasurer, secretary). One could participate in AHIMA-related surveys, focus groups, or be a coding roundtable coordinator. Mentoring opportunities abound, as well as writing and/or speaking engagements.

AHIMA Advocacy Center

AHIMA has an advocacy and public policy center online for members to access for multiple purposes. The Advocacy Agenda is available for reading. The agenda advances HIM practices primarily for the purpose of improving the effectiveness of the electronic health record (EHR) throughout the healthcare realm. The agenda has identified several priorities related to AHIMA's overall vision. These priorities are EHR adoption, health information exchange (HIE), privacy and security of health information, clinical documentation improvement (CDI), HIM workforce, and HIM recognition. The advocacy site has resources available for members to research elected officials and legislative issues through the Advocacy Assistant.

Change Management

Change management

Change is the only constant in a work environment. Change is inevitable. In fact, change is guaranteed in life. People handle change differently—some embrace it, while others resist it. Change management is a necessary component of personnel management. Change management can be defined as a structured approach of ensuring that changes are implemented successfully and smoothly, and are sustainable (meaning the benefits of change last). It is important to note that change is not isolated to one person, but rather it affects many people, whether the effect is only intradepartmental related or related to the organization as a whole. Objectives of change management may include: active support from administration or senior managers; involvement of key individuals to oversee the implementation of the changes; determining the impact of the changes on staff; effective open communication to all involved; and, effective staff training prior to, during, and after implementation to ensure all involved are thoroughly prepared for the changes.

Selecting new EHR or CAC vendors

Successful implementation of a new EHR or CAC system involves several key steps. The planning process is always imperative to the success of the project. This step helps the healthcare entity determine what, when, and how to identify funding and necessary resources. The budgeting aspect of this step includes costs related to the purchase of the software as well as its associated installation and maintenance fees. Following planning, vendor selection and the implementation phase would occur. Choosing the vendor would be based on which one best meets the needs of the organization. The implementation phase would involve an analysis of workflows, documentation review, and data storage. Staff training would be the next step in the implementation of a new system. Effective training measures will result in employees who walk away with a high level of confidence in the new system and the role they assume in using the product(s). After go-live, it would be necessary to monitor and analyze workflow processes to measure productivity, assess quality of work, determine whether further education is needed, and provide return on investment data to administration.

Challenges of HIM consolidations

Centralization or consolidation of HIM services between healthcare entities or through healthcare mergers is quite commonplace in today's healthcare landscape. These consolidations are occurring primarily secondary to shifting reimbursement methodologies, which are affecting healthcare costs. In other words, the cost of healthcare services is out of control, and hospitals and physician offices/clinics are forced to find ways to save money, and in many cases, the best solution is to merge with other healthcare entities. When healthcare mergers occur, multiple challenges arise primarily due to disparate systems. Examples of challenges include reduction in staff force, logistics of healthcare locations (e.g., long distances apart, making it difficult to transport documents), staffing schedule adjustments, learning curve related to new systems and/or workflow processes, new or unexpected costs, and physician reaction to changes in HIM services.

Problem-solving measures

Centralization or consolidation of HIM services between healthcare entities or through healthcare mergers is quite commonplace in today's healthcare landscape. With the mergers, HIM professionals face multiple challenges, and for these challenges it is important to be aware of problem-solving techniques necessary to counter the challenges. For example, HIM professionals should work collaboratively with employees from all levels. Collaborative communication is the key to success of the mergers. If possible, steps should be taken to retain staff from rural hospitals whose departments are being merged into larger hospital settings. Allowing work from remote locations should be given ample consideration. It is important to understand the needs and concerns of all HIM departments involved in the merger, and then ensure that those needs and concerns are proactively addressed. Be transparent with staff as much as possible, outlining for them goals, objectives, and expectations. Finally, it is important during a merger to work closely with physicians, keeping them informed of the merger's progress or lack of progress, and requesting their feedback and input.

Work Design & Process Improvement

Implementing productivity standards

With the recent implementation of ICD-10 as of October 1, 2015 and regular updates as of October 1, 2016, there are several methods to consider for implementation pertaining to productivity standards. These methods include the following:

- Monitor the average coding time per record and trend the results. Initially, the average coding time would have increased in comparison to ICD-9 average coding times; however, over time, the average coding times in ICD-10 should begin to decrease.
- Monitor coding productivity by the case mix index (CMI). Coding productivity, for those coders working in cases with a high CMI, would be longer than those with a low CMI.
- Assess the average coding time for the top 25 DRGs for the designated entity.

Once these results are monitored and trended over a select period of time, productivity standards can be developed because these measures help to identify codes and/or DRGs for which it takes a longer period of time to complete.

Establishment of coding productivity standards

The formula to calculate a coder's production is simple: Subtract the hours of non-coding tasks (also known as "downtime") from the total hours of coding tasks. Of note, non-coding tasks should include education/training, system technical problems, data analysis projects, etc. Then divide the number of accounts coded by the hours spent coding. This will provide the number of accounts coded per hour. This formula can be built into database functions, available for the coder and manager to acknowledge. This formula may be easy, but there are other factors to consider when determining the coder's overall skill level. For example, quality of work or coding accuracy must be monitored, striving to reach or surpass the national standard of 95% coding accuracy.

Designing electronic HIM workflow processes

When designing an electronic HIM workflow, it is important to first understand basic workflow logic. One step in a workflow process can perform multiple actions if designed to do so. Workflow processes should be designed so that they flow logically from the previous step. If a step in the flow contains only actions and no conditions, then the workflow will perform the designated actions. If a

- 68 -

step includes conditions, then the step can only be satisfied when the conditions are met. A workflow must be hyperlinked or attached to a preexisting database, list, or library, and if there are no preexisting resources, then a new resource must be created. To complete a newly designed workflow, the final step is to test the process before publishing, and if an error exists (such as a break in a hyperlink), then error symbols will appear next to each step for the parameter that is invalid. Measures will then need to be taken to correct the errors.

Workflows

Workflow is the logical progression of steps for the purpose of accomplishing tasks, through the process of passing along data or information to a participant for further action, in compliance with pre-established procedural rules. Healthcare organizations use workflows to coordinate tasks between individuals or departments and ultimately accomplish procedural efficiency, procedural compliance, cost savings, and transparency (through visible audit trails). There are basically 3 different types of workflows: sequential workflow (similar to flowcharts), state machine workflow (more complex, returning to a previous step if needed), and rules-driven workflow (the rules determine the progress of the workflow). Workflow software (eg, SharePoint) offer many benefits, such as improved productivity, transparency, faster turnaround times, improved accountability, cost savings, and reduction in error rates.

Workflow analysis

Workflow analysis is the process of reviewing all steps in a workflow to identify inefficiencies and then recommend improvement opportunities. The analysis process involves meeting with "owners" of the workflow to gain an understanding of their current process, any known problems/issues, and their desired outcome. Continuous process improvement should be sought by healthcare entities, especially in light of technological advancements and constant change. Workflow analysis can take into account these changes and make recommendations on how to improve workflows to be more efficient and less costly. A large portion of workflow analysis includes interviewing key individuals involved in the workflow. This includes those who are involved at the beginning of the workflow process and extends to those at the end of the workflow. Documentation of each workflow step is key to identifying inefficiencies and identifying opportunities for improvement. Once the analysis is completed, the results are typically presented to lower-level management to ensure that the results are accurate and realistic. After adjustments are made, the final recommendations are made to administration for their consideration.

Process improvement plan

Process improvement plans should include the following components:

- An abstract or summary of the overall plan
- Approvals by responsible parties
- Revision history of the plan to include the revision number, release date, author's name, and reason for change(s)
- Purpose of the document
- Definitions of key terms, acronyms, and abbreviations
- Cited references or resources
- Plan overview to include the scope, goals, and objectives
- Key stakeholders and their roles and responsibilities in the project
- Critical success factors
- Assumptions about the plan

- 69 -

- Constraints of the plan
- Risks that may have a negative impact on the plan
- Tracking of risks and issues and logs pertaining to the risks and issues
- Status reporting throughout the various phases of the plan
- Implementation phase to introduce the project to the organization
- Training requirements
- Project deliverables and repository
- Project schedule and key milestones.

Human Resources Management

Staff recruitment

In the health information field, disparities exist between new graduates and experienced professionals. Finding credentialed, experienced staff can be a difficult process, but strategies can be used to find the best candidates. The strategies include:

- Effective communication between HIM professionals and human resource (HR) personnel. It is the HIM professional's responsibility to inform the HR rep of how a vacancy is impacting the health system's bottom line.
- Competitive compensation is key to successful recruitment. The compensation benefits may go beyond salary to include the potential benefits of a flexible schedule, working remotely, relocation expenses, etc.
- Proactive recruiting is an important strategy for staff recruitment and may include networking through professional organizations, using state professional organization sites to post job vacancies free of charge, and offering bonuses to current employees for referrals.

Creating HIM job descriptions

The process of creating an HIM job description should begin with a job analysis. The purpose of a job analysis is to determine what skills, knowledge, and abilities are required of the employee. The job analysis allows management the opportunity to establish authority (reporting lines) and determine measures of performance. Once the job analysis is completed, a job description can be created. The description should identify duties and responsibilities for a certain job, physical expectations (eg, standing, eyesight), work environment layout, and reporting structure. It is important to note that the job description should be the resource document for performance evaluations.

Progressive disciplinary action

When managing employees, it is inevitable that there will be times when expected results are not achieved by an employee, and this failure warrants disciplinary action. It is recommended that the formal system of disciplinary action be followed, and assistance from an HR rep should be requested. A formal system of disciplinary action includes verbal warnings, written warnings, suspension, and termination. The formal system should include a list of minor versus major issues with minor issues typically resolved through a verbal warning, written warning, or suspension. Examples of a written warning may be unsatisfactory performance or attendance issues. Major problems can result in immediate termination, such as theft or intoxication on the job. With any form of disciplinary action, documentation should always be maintained. It is reasonable to involve 2 managers in the conversations held with the employee for an extra level of protection against unjust accusations.

Training & Development

Effective training for providers

Effective training platforms for hospital-affiliated providers should be conducted with the understanding that providers are interested in the patient-care perspective more so than the coding classification system. Physician education sessions should be provided as continuing medical education opportunities, and the goal should be to inform the provider of how effective documentation practices will affect his/her quality outcomes and pay-for-performance initiatives. Departmental medical staff meetings or quarterly staff meetings are excellent opportunities to cover documentation improvement practices. One-on-one educational sessions tend to be the best approach because the department's own documentation practices can be highlighted. The intervention of a physician advisor in educational efforts is an effective approach to improving documentation practices because the communication is peer-to-peer and better received. Coding roundtables are educational sessions that focus on coding, data analysis, and documentation improvement topics. This can be an opportunity for coders, clinical documentation improvement (CDI) specialists, and physicians to collaborate and discuss opportunities for process change.

Continuing education regarding healthcare privacy

Training for providers regarding privacy is not optional for healthcare entities. The Health Insurance Portability and Accountability Act (HIPAA) requires that all staff (including contracted individuals and volunteers) must be trained in maintaining the privacy and confidentiality of protected health information. The training must be provided to new staff members within a reasonable time of their employment date (e.g., employers provide the training as part of on-boarding of new staff members). Documentation that training occurred must be maintained for each staff member. Policies and procedures (P&Ps) pertaining to privacy and confidentiality must be kept current, and when changes are made to the P&Ps, subsequent training must be carried out. Confidentiality/privacy training must be conducted annually for all employees in order to keep employees up-to-date with current privacy practices.

Effective orientation process

Orientation is the process of providing relevant information to a new employee so that he/she is well informed/equipped to perform his/her job responsibilities with as much ease as possible in the beginning. Orientation goals and objectives should be outlined prior to the first day of employment, and then used as a reference tool to guide the manager and the new employee through the orientation period. The new employee should be oriented to the department space and equipment functions and storage, as well as be introduced to employees relevant to the success of his/her job. All relevant paperwork should be completed during this time frame, including confidentiality acknowledgements. Employee handbooks or relevant policies and procedures should be provided to the new staff member, and a sufficient amount of time to review the material should be allowed. Work schedules should be determined, if not agreed on prior to employment, and clock-in/clock-out procedures should be reviewed. It is important to not overload the new employee with too much information, but rather present materials over time. It is important to use an orientation checklist to ensure that all necessary information has been provided. This will provide evidence that all aspects of employment were reviewed with the new employee, in the event of any future claims pertaining to human resource noncompliance.

Designing an effective training program

An effective training program will only be successful when the time and effort is made to design a solid framework beginning with a preliminary needs assessment and analysis and ending with an evaluation. Needs assessment and analysis includes asking pertinent questions, such as "Is a training session needed, or is distribution of written communication enough to address the educational goals and objectives?" It is important to be clear about the organizational or departmental needs and the expected or desired business results. Once the needs assessment is completed, the scope, audience, and resources available should be identified or designated, along with the learning objectives and measurement methods. The method of delivering the training should be determined at this point (e.g., online, webinars, classroom, PowerPoint, other templates) as well as the materials needed (e.g., quick reference guides, dry erase boards or flip charts, paper, posters, writing tools). At this point in the design process, the instructor(s) should be selected, keeping in mind that the instructor will be instrumental in whether the training is successful. A test run or pilot training session is helpful to assess any weak areas. Once corrected, the training sessions should be conducted, and then completed with evaluation opportunities for future consideration of changes needed.

Effective methods of teaching adult learners

Adults learn using a variety of different methods. Interactive methods are effective ways for adults to best comprehend the material because it allows the adult learner to apply knowledge into a situation or realistic scenario. In addition to selecting the educational delivery method, the instructor must understand all students will possess varying comprehension levels. It is always best to present information on an eighth-grade comprehension level. Examples of effective interactive methods to use are role play, brainstorming, demonstration, and tours. Role-playing case scenarios provide opportunities to experience relationship issues in a work environment. Brainstorming methods allow for creative ideas and/or solutions to be shared. Demonstrative methods by the instructor reveal the step-by-step procedure(s) for job functions, and can be followed with a time for the student to repeat the newly learned process. Tours of work areas allow students the opportunity to visualize a job in process as well as contact with individuals who may be able to answer questions from by the students.

Attributes of effective teachers

Teachers/Instructors are instrumental in enhancing the learning experience. A variety of methods promote effective teaching. For example, effective teachers will possess great organizational skills. They will understand the importance of using clear and simple explanations and examples, as well as a variety of instructional materials and learning activities. Effective delivery of information will be presented at multiple cognitive levels. The effective teacher will offer many opportunities to the students to elaborate on their insights, so that higher critical thinking skills are achieved. A passion for teaching as well as being a subject matter expert are attributes of effective teachers. Encouragement and praise are frequently offered by exceptional teachers.

Strategic & Organizational Management

Current HIM trends

The healthcare environment is constantly changing, with multiple opportunities for health care and the HIM profession, but risks as well. A scan of the healthcare environment, and specifically how opportunities and risks are affecting the HIM profession, has identified the following trends:

technology advancements, cloud services, big data, mobile health, consumer control of health information, and the growth of health information exchange. Technology advancements continue to reinvent the delivery of health care, and in terms of how technology has affected health information management, the power of data has opened opportunities for information access and the development of new reimbursement models. Cloud services are being used to host health information applications. Big data is increasing opportunities for HIM professionals to participate in clinical informatics and/or data analysts. Mobile health services (eg, smart phones and tablets) are changing the landscape of healthcare delivery. Use of apps to track patient information as well as operationalize physician practices brings many opportunities for healthcare improvement as well as challenges. Consumers desire more control of their health information through online access, and as a result health information exchange use is growing exponentially.

Using audits to monitor organizational needs

The Code of Federal Regulations (CFR) has published a standard that mandates that covered entities must have audit controls in place to monitor information systems that contain electronic patient health information. This standard does not outline the audit process, and as a result, healthcare entities tend to react to organizational processes/needs/issues, rather than proactively monitor them. Regardless of whether the audit process is reactive or proactive, the primary concern is to ensure that audits are conducted to identify organizational risks and needs. The audit process should include identification of who will be audited, which systems will be audited, the audit frequency, and reporting of audit findings in conjunction with educational efforts to correct noncompliant findings.

Current trends in healthcare data

The role of a health information data analyst continues to evolve as the world of electronic health records matures. In this present electronic age, healthcare data (whether clinically, administratively, or financially related) are limitless. The following data trends represent the limitless opportunities of health information management:

- Calculation of patient wait times to be seen by a healthcare provider
- Calculation of readmission rates (which can have a significant financial impact)
- Monitoring of complication and/or mortality rates
- Monitoring of public health data
- Monitoring the average length of stay
- Analysis of patient quality scores.

This list is not exhaustive. Trending these data sets will tell a story, upon which the healthcare entity can make important healthcare decisions (administratively, clinically, and financially) moving forward.

Trending coding compliance data

Healthcare administration will expect to receive information (daily, monthly, or quarterly) pertaining to coding compliance. Each healthcare entity will need to decide what coding compliance data should be collected, the frequency of its collection, and the reasoning behind its collection. This should be acknowledged through policies and procedures. The importance of collecting and trending coding compliance data is understood to impact (either directly or indirectly) clinical and financial decision making. Examples of coding compliance data that should be collected are (this list is not exhaustive):

- DRG assignment accuracy
- Present on admission (POA) indicator assignment accuracy
- Discharge disposition assignment accuracy
- Principal diagnosis code assignment accuracy
- Principal procedure code assignment accuracy
- Validation of attending physician and surgeon names assigned in the abstract
- Coding and/or auditing productivity.

Measuring the productivity of coding audits, the coding compliance accuracy rates, and the associated overall net financial impact can be used in a cost benefit analysis to support additional staff acquisitions. For example, if 2 coding auditors yield a net financial impact (based on DRG changes resulting from the audits) of $1 million annually, then further calculations can be conducted to illustrate the projected monetary gain if more coding auditors were hired.

Cost-benefit analysis

A cost-benefit analysis is a detailed financial outline pertaining to a proposal or project. Typically, a cost-benefit analysis will project a financial impact based on literal costs. Itemization of projected costs is a necessary component. Projected costs may be a one-time cost (e.g., purchase of a software package) or an ongoing expense (e.g., projected salaries). Not only should projections be reflective of tangible costs but also intangible costs, such as the cost of time spent away from normal job responsibilities in order to complete the project, energy costs associated with the project, and costs associated with changing routine schedules. In addition to analyzing projected costs associated with the project, benefits should be considered as well. Benefits may include projected financial gain, monetary savings, as well as time savings associated with improved workflow. The final step in a cost-benefit analysis is to determine the total costs and compare if the projected benefits substantiate the projected costs. Ultimately, management needs to know whether a project is profitable and feasible.

Business planning

A business plan is a strategic effort to describe the future of a business or service, and how the plan for its success will be achieved. It entails the development of a vision, goals, and objectives, and identification of resources and abilities. The key content of the plan should include marketing strategies, competitive analyses, design and development of services, financial factors, as well as the operations and management of the business. The value of a business plan lies in seeing things realistically. This reality can only be attained after one has examined the market for a particular service, identified potential customers (eg, patients in health care), determined the team makeup, and identified a business model to follow. In health care, business planning takes the same elements described above and focuses them on health care services and patients. In such a plan, the following should be assessed: healthcare trends, service types per patient types (eg, home health services for elderly patients), healthcare software (eg, EHR, reimbursement models), and patient population statistics in order to determine the patient volume that could be served annually.

Management of business associate agreements

In health care, contractual agreements are made between the healthcare entity and business associates. These business associates are responsible for ensuring the security and privacy of electronic patient health information (ePHI) as the healthcare provider. In other words, HIPAA regulations do apply to any business associate (e.g., software vendors, clearinghouses) who creates, receives, maintains, or transmits ePHI. These transactions are referenced as "satisfactory assurances" under HIPAA and the HITECH Act of 2009. The business associate agreement (BAA) must comply with the regulations in the following ways: business associates must implement safeguards to protect PHI (e.g., prevent unauthorized disclosures). The business associate must provide to the Department of Health and Human Services (HHS) a copy of their policies and procedures pertaining to HIPAA compliance. At termination of a BAA, the business associate must return to the healthcare provider all PHI or destroy all PHI. The business associate must agree to hold any subcontractors to the same HIPAA standards. All BAA contracts should be audited/assessed for compliance regarding privacy, security, financial obligations, and other regulatory components.

Capital budget

A capital budget can be defined as a plan that shows major expenditures and identifies the resources of funding to support the expenditures. Healthcare capital budget items may include medical equipment, facilities/buildings, land, transportation, etc. Capital expenditures will impact services for a period extending beyond a year. Capital expenses will include a total investment that exceeds monetary values preestablished by the medical board. Capital expenses must be justified for the board's review and approval or disapproval. Justification of a capital budget should include the following: reason for the capital expenditure request, options or alternatives to the request, proposal containing detailed information, benefit analysis, cost analysis, prioritization of expenses, and time frame phases.

Financial Management

Personnel budget process

The personnel budget is an important expense budget process. It involves forecasting staffing needs as well as departmental and organizational trends. In health care, fluctuations in admission/discharge rates can affect staffing needs, as well as external regulatory changes that may affect workloads (e.g., RAC requests). It is important for HIM professionals to monitor productivity measures throughout the fiscal year in order to make accurate personnel projections. Tools may be used to assist with staffing calculations, such as Excel spreadsheets. Data to be collected on the spreadsheets may be hourly wage/salary, exempt/non-exempt status, projected annual hours of work, projected annual overtime hours of work, projected cost of living raises or merit increases, and estimated non-productivity time (e.g., vacation time, sick leave, FMLA). It is beneficial to compare the upcoming fiscal year's personnel staffing proposal with the current year's budget and even the previous year's budget.

Operating budget process

The operating budget is known as the non-wage or non-salary expense budget. It encapsulates all other costs associated with the revenue and expense budget process. Typical categories pertaining to an operating budget may include literature, contractual services, forms/paper materials, travel, membership dues, minor equipment, office supplies, printing inhouse, professional fees, postage, repair services, and storage. In development of an operating expense budget, it is necessary to determine the unit of service for each expense type as well as its associated cost (variable versus fixed). Variable expenses are more difficult to determine as they depend on vendors, rate of inflation, supply costs, etc. Fixed expenses are easier to project as they are usually a one-time

- 75 -

purchase, such as minor equipment. It is beneficial for management to monitor expenses and unit costs throughout the year in order to determine cost variances and make any necessary adjustments so that the budget is not exceeded.

Budget variance

A budget variance can be defined as the difference between what was projected to be the cost and what was actually the cost. Naturally, a budget variance is favorable when the actual expenditure is less than the budgeted amount. In other words, the budget variance improves the net financial income. Budget variances occur when budget assumptions are not reasonable or over/under estimated. Budget variances tend to happen when unexpected expenses (such as equipment repair) or unpredictable events (e.g., a natural disaster that creates water damage) occur. It is important to not be too overly optimistic in the budgeting process or base budget decisions on too few facts or data, as these scenarios often lead to budget variances. When budget variances occur, management should investigate the root cause.

Analysis

A budget variance analysis is simple. It is the review of a budget to assess if the financial income is under or over the budget or if the budget was met. It is a time of reflection on accuracy of budget projections as well as root cause analysis of overexpenditures. Variances will either be favorable or adverse for the healthcare organization. It is best to use percentage calculations to determine the net financial impact. The accounting formula to use is: %Budget Variance = (Actual - Budget)/Budget. Administration will expect an explanation of the budget variance analysis. Management will need to communicate effectively the budget accuracies and inaccuracies. Examples of consequences may include: restrictions on travel, restrictions on educational opportunities, hiring freezes, or decreased funding for costs in the upcoming fiscal year.

Budget benchmarking

Budget benchmarking is a technique in which a healthcare entity may compare its budget results with its own performance in previous years, or the entity may compare its budget results with another healthcare entity, or the entity may compare its budget results with professional organizational standards. By comparing against its own historical performance, an organization can assess its previous revenue and expenses and make sound judgments for the upcoming fiscal year. Conducting a comparison against another healthcare entity requires a concerted effort. Finding an institution willing to share the information can be difficult, and once a willing participant is discovered, it requires time to interview management and determine how their financial experience compares with the organization seeking assistance. It is important to determine upfront the level of internal performance that is desired; is it acceptable to have cost control or does this healthcare entity desire to be the forerunner in financial finesse. Finally, to compare budget results against professional organization standards can be quite beneficial. Professional standards may include financial measures to confirm financial stability as well as cost control.

Ethics

AHIMA's Code of Ethics

Purpose

The American Health Information Management Association is a professional organization that has established ethical obligations. These ethical obligations, also known as the Code of Ethics, primarily pertains to the creation, use, and maintenance of health information; the safeguarding of privacy and security of health information; and the accessibility and integrity of health information. This Code of Ethics guides the conduct of HIM professionals who hold AHIMA credentials and/or Commission on Certification for Health Informatics and Information Management (CCHIIM) credentials. This Code of Ethics promotes the integrity of the organization and ultimately helps to improve the overall quality of health care. The AHIMA Code of Ethics supports 7 purposes: high health information standards, established core values, broad ethical principles, guides for decision making, framework for professional behavior and responsibilities, accountability standards, and mentoring principles. The code is designed to be a reference to enforce or encourage professional ethical behavior.

Principles

AHIMA's Code of Ethics is subdivided into a list of 11 ethical principles based on AHIMA's core values. In addition, guidelines enhance the ethical principles in order to provide clarification. The principles are applicable to all certified AHIMA members. Briefly, the 11 ethical principles can be summarized as follows:

- Advocate privacy and confidentiality
- Promote integrity and professionalism in the work environment by showing honor to others
- Advocate security of health information
- Refuse participation in unethical practices
- Participate in continuing education to stay current in HIM practices
- Develop and strengthen the HIM professional workforce
- Be a positive HIM representative
- Perform associational responsibilities with integrity
- Represent credentials truthfully
- Facilitate collaboration of interdisciplinary relationships
- Show respect to all people.

Guidelines associated with principles

Principle	Summary of Guideline Examples
Advocate privacy and confidentiality.	All protected health information must be kept confidential, and rights to privacy must be followed.
Promote integrity and professionalism in the work environment by showing honor to others.	Maintain a state of professionalism at all times by promoting integrity, trust, and service to others.
Advocate security of health information.	Health information (regardless of medium) must be protected and preserved. Inappropriate disclosure and access must be avoided.
Refuse participation in unethical practices.	Discourage and correct unethical behavior when necessary.
Participate in continuing education to stay current in HIM practices.	Pursue opportunities to become subject matter experts of HIM knowledge.
Develop and strengthen the HIM professional workforce.	Provide and/or participate in educational opportunities through directed practice or mentoring to build the HIM workforce.
Be a positive HIM representative.	Promote the HIM profession; be an advocate.
Perform associational responsibilities with integrity.	Operate and adhere to the associational bylaws, fulfilling responsibilities of an associational position.

Represent credentials truthfully.	Represent professional qualifications to others accurately.
Facilitate collaboration of interdisciplinary relationships.	Promote collaborative efforts between healthcare disciplines for the benefit of the patient.
Show respect to all people.	Promote the value of each person.

Consequences of violating the Code of Ethics

Violation of AHIMA's Code of Ethics by a credentialed professional may be addressed by legal procedures or subjected to a peer review process. The peer review process is typically separate from any legal proceedings. The purpose of the peer review process is to give the opportunity for the organization to counsel and/or discipline ethical noncompliance. Violations, however, may warrant legal action when federal or state regulations are disregarded. The Code of Ethics is not a list of rules that describes behaviors in all health information management activities. To understand the application of the code, consider the context of each standard/principle before determining conflicts and associated consequences.

Project Management

Project management

Project management can be defined as the assessment of project requirements and the implementation of necessary activities to achieve the requirements. For a project to be successfully managed, the responsible individual(s) will need to use knowledge, experience, skills, and tools. These elements for projective management success are exhibited through leadership experience, effective communication skills, conflict management experience, critical thinking skills, and effective problem-solving skills. Tools often used by project managers may be Microsoft Project, Excel, PowerPoint, OneNote, or cloud-based tools. Sharing information, plans, and resources among project team members is essential to success. The phases of project management are initiation, planning, implementation, monitoring, and completion. Project initiation includes the development of a vision along with goals and objectives and stakeholder support. Planning takes into account budget requirements, schedules, assigned responsibilities, etc. Implementation will involve resource management, quality assurance, and team approach. Monitoring will focus on identifying and quantifying variances, and the completion will identify if the project scope was accomplished.

Healthcare project manager's role

A healthcare project manager should possess management skills, technical knowledge, and project management tool experience (eg, Access, Excel, PowerPoint, Visio). Leadership skills are necessary as well, specifically in the following areas: diversity, in terms of working with multiple team members from different backgrounds; visionary, in terms of clearly outlining goals and objectives as well as alterative plans; teamwork, for the purpose of building relationships and trust; conflict resolution to ensure poor relationships or ineffective communication does not hinder progress; influence, to ensure activities stay on schedule and are accomplished. The project manager will be responsible for encouraging collaboration in the face of challenges and conflict. This person is also responsible for identifying alternative options or intelligent solutions when resistance to current goals, objectives, or activities is encountered.

Project charter

A project charter is typically a 1-page document that sets the vision and/or the boundaries for the project. The charter will include the project name and its description, the key stakeholders involved in the project (e.g., manager, team members), cost-benefit analysis, projected budget, projected time frame from beginning to conclusion, and administrative authorization to proceed with the project. It serves as the foundation or framework of the project. Each of these elements or phases are further defined or elaborated on in separate documents or forums. The charter serves as the starting point of the project.

Project scope

The scope of a project sets boundaries. It determines what elements are included and not included in the project. Without boundaries, "scope creep" can occur, which is a subtle process of continuous growth that ultimately results in not meeting project goals or not finishing on time. It is important to develop a scope statement that identifies a detailed description of products or services expected to be delivered, proposed project steps, and definitions of what projects and/or services will be considered successful. The scope will need to be broken down into a detailed representation of the expected deliverable (product or service), the activity to achieve the deliverable, the responsible party, and the success criteria. An example of how this may appear might be:

Deliverable	Activity	Success Criteria
Electronic dashboard of coding accuracy data	Identify valid coding data resources	Coding data resources are validated as reliable during 100% of testing phase.

Once the scope statement is determined, key stakeholders should sign off on it in order to "freeze" the scope. Then, when changes develop as the project progresses, the changes must go through a formal process of approval or disapproval.

Time management

Time management is a critical element of project management. One effective time management tool to use is a network diagram. The network diagram illustrates the sequence of project events/activities. It should demonstrate for each activity the number of expected days to completion. For example, activity 1 (identify valid coding data resources) may be assigned a total of 2 days to complete. This illustration develops a timeline or a Gantt chart (a popular tool used by project managers). The Gantt chart provides a detailed explanation of the various activities, the beginning and ending dates, the length of time scheduled for each activity, and where activities might overlap. Inevitably, there are activities that will have a longer path to completion than others. Longer paths are known as critical paths because they tend to delay progress. It is important for the project manager to focus on the critical paths in order to investigate root causes of the delays and implement actions to move ahead.

Vendor/Contract Management

Vendor contract

Contractual agreements between a healthcare entity and a vendor may take the form of either a fixed price contract, a time and material contract, or a hybrid contract. A fixed price contract will be based on an agreement of a fixed fee for the product or service. A time and material contract is an agreement based on a fee rate wherein the vendor bills the healthcare entity for actual materials and time involved. A hybrid contract is a mixture of the two and tends to be more complex. The typical elements of any contract include scope, goal, objectives, deliverables, and legal terms and conditions. Establishing the scope is important because it prevents misunderstandings later on. It will be necessary for the healthcare entity to identify all objectives during this phase of the agreement. Software, equipment, communication, data backup, and archiving needs should all be determined in this negotiation stage, as well as what services will be provided after termination of the contract (eg, access to archived data). Detailed description of deliverables is a critical element of negotiation. The extent of services or products provided should be negotiated (eg, life of equipment, replacement fees, maintenance fees).

Contract reviews

Contract reviews by corporate compliance officials are increasingly important in health care. This is primarily due to federal and/or state regulations pertaining to reimbursement, Medicare/Medicaid, Stark Law, and other areas of increased scrutiny by the Office of Inspector General (OIG). Healthcare contractual agreements are developed with vendors, physician groups, clinical services (e.g., long-term dialysis arrangements), and post-acute care arrangements (e.g., hospice, rehab, skilled nursing). When reviewing these types of contracts, compliance experts need to focus on the following:

- Professional qualifications/credentials
- Scheduled hours of provider-based coverage
- Financial arrangements to include billing, reimbursement, and/or compensation based on fair market value
- Adherence to anti-kickback statutes
- Potential conflict of interest issues
- Code of conduct terms
- Adherence to the healthcare facility's policies and procedures
- Ownership and retention of information.

Safeguards to consider when outsourcing coding services

Coding shortages exist in the United States, and to compensate for the shortage, many healthcare entities seek assistance through outsourcing. Outsourcing of coding services may stay within the United States, but due to less expensive costs, many healthcare entities choose off-shore services. Regardless of the external corporation selected for the outsourced coding services, it is imperative the healthcare entity consider certain negotiating questions for the contracting company. These negotiating points of discovery should include, at a minimum, the following:

- Adherence to HIPAA standards
- Adherence to all federal and/or state regulations
- Adherence to information security practices
- Assurance of financial stability
- Professional experience to compliantly meet coding standards
- Efficient and effective transfer of data between operating systems
- Identified risks of outsourcing.

Enterprise Information Management

Strategic planning

Financial perspective

When involved in strategic planning, an HIM professional should examine the current business/economic trends. This would include analyzing budget constraints, data integrity, efficiency requirements, reimbursement changes, and the lack of funding for regulatory mandates. Budget constraints are inevitable secondary to rising healthcare costs. HIM departments will need to support budget requests by showing a return on investment. Data integrity is important in financial strategic planning because quality data is increasingly used to support financial models. Efficiency in work performance is more desirable in today's healthcare environment because of budget constraints and reimbursement changes. Staff will be expected to possess more skills and more flexibility in job performance. Reimbursement changes occur annually whether through federal payers decreasing reimbursement or through the advent of newly developed reimbursement models (e.g., accountable care organizations). Lack of funding for legislative mandates (e.g., recovery audit contractor audits) requires strategic planning skills for the HIM professional as well.

Demographic perspective

When involved in strategic planning, an HIM professional should examine the current demographic trends. Pertinent demographic trends that require strategic planning by the HIM professional include topics such as aging AHIMA membership, globalization of information, lack of volunteers, and offshore employees. Because of the changing HIM landscape, it is estimated that new HIM jobs far outreach the number of HIM professionals available to fill the vacancies. This requires an awareness by the seasoned HIM professional when trying to find experienced employees (eg, inexperienced employees with sufficient training methods should be pursued). The availability of information globally allows numerous opportunities for education and exchange of new ideas in the health information field. Virtual collaboration can be a viable means to strategically plan. Strategic planning will be necessary when it comes to fulfilling associational membership activities. Decreased volunteerism due to organizations' unwillingness to allow time for participation in associational activities makes it more difficult to manage member involvement. Outsourcing of HIM jobs due to economic constraints will require strategic planning as well, particularly in relation to controlling costs and ensuring quality of services.

Legislative perspective

With the growth of federal and state regulations, healthcare entities are heavily burdened to ensure compliance with legislation (such as the Affordable Care Act). Strategic planning by HIM professionals is a necessity. Affordable care organizations (ACOs) are being developed at a fast pace, and this requires strategic planning pertaining to information exchange as well as data integrity. Big data impacting health care is overwhelmingly burdensome to HIM professionals. HIM professionals, being information experts, are key to embracing big data and learning how to use it efficiently and meaningfully. Electronic transmission of health information is evolving rapidly and requires HIM insight for effective strategic planning. Not only have federal payers moved to tying payments to quality performance, but private payers are following suit. This requires HIM professionals to strategically consider the shift in incentives from volume-based methods to now quality of care and/or health-focused value.

Technology perspective

Technological advances keep HIM professionals in a strategic planning state of mind. Communication mediums are numerous and are revolutionizing the HIM field. Portable devices, apps, and social media all bring a new perspective on how to protect health information. Use of computer-assisted coding (CAC) software is growing and requires strategic planning in terms of its effectiveness, accuracy, and efficiency. A key part of CAC is natural language processing (NLP), which is built into CAC and other aspects of electronic health records (EHRs). HIM professionals will need to strategically consider their impact on health care. Health information exchange (HIE) should be an element of strategic planning as well. Its growth is exponential, and concerns regarding data privacy, security, timeliness, completeness, and accuracy should be an area of focus.

RHIA Practice Test

1. What type of data does the Atlas Severity of Illness System present?

    a. ordinal
    b. nominal
    c. continuous
    d. discrete

2. In which type of health maintenance organization do all of the providers work in the same facility?

    a. group model
    b. network type
    c. independent practice association
    d. staff model

3. Which of the following are NOT a component of a PERT network?

    a. activities
    b. events
    c. goals
    d. reasons

4. Which of the following is a characteristic of the terminal digit filing system?

    a. The training period is relatively short.
    b. All inactive files are pulled from the same area.
    c. Each number is divided into pairs of digits.
    d. Files tend to expand at the back end of the number series.

5. During the month of March, a healthcare facility sees 140 total cases and provides service with a total value of 179. What is the case mix index for this period? Round your answer to the nearest tenth.

    a. 0.4
    b. 0.8
    c. 1.3
    d. 1.8

6. A healthcare facility had 3000 discharges (including deaths) and 35 nosocomial infections. What was the nosocomial infection rate for the facility? Round your answer to the nearest tenth of a percent.

    a. 1.2%
    b. 9.4%
    c. 47.2%
    d. 85.7%

7. Which coding instrument is generally recommended for principal diagnosis upon admittance to inpatient treatment?

    a. SNOMED
    b. ICD-9-CM
    c. DSM-5
    d. HCPCS

8. Which of the following is NOT a feature of automated record tracking systems?

a. Staff members receive an alert when a file is returned while they are away.
b. Requests are prioritized manually.
c. Multiple file room locations can be tracked.
d. These systems are updated in real time.

9. During the month of April, the pediatrics department of a hospital sees 25 patients. Their average length of stay is three days. The internal medicine department sees 50 patients. Their average length of stay is four days. What is the weighted average length of stay for the month of April? Round your answer to the nearest tenth.

a. 0.5 days
b. 3.7 days
c. 4.4 days
d. 5.4 days

10. Which financial statement provides a snapshot of a company's position at a specific time?

a. income statement
b. balance sheet
c. statement of owner's equity
d. statement of cash flows

11. A study focuses on determining the proportion of patients with dental problems whose care plans adhere to the American Dental Association's guidelines. Which dimension of performance is addressed by this study?

a. efficacy
b. appropriateness
c. continuity
d. efficiency

12. Which organization maintains the Central Office on ICD-9-CM?

a. National Center for Health Statistics
b. American Hospital Association
c. American Health Information Management Association
d. Health Care Financing Administration

13. A blood pressure measurement is an example of which of the following types of data?

a. continuous
b. discrete
c. nominal
d. ordinal

14. Which Medicare reimbursement methodology is used in physician offices and clinics?

a. prospective payment system per diem
b. ambulatory surgery center groups
c. prospective payment system based on diagnosis-related groups
d. resources-based relative value system

15. What is the mode of the data set below?

(1, 4, 6, 6, 8, 9, 12, 15, 18)

    a. 1
    b. 6
    c. 8
    d. 15

16. For the month of July, the case mix value of a particular diagnosis-related group was 1.4, and 40 cases were recorded. What was the total value of service for July? Round your answer to the nearest whole number.

    a. 22
    b. 29
    c. 37
    d. 56

17. Which data item is LEAST likely to appear on the clinical forms of a patient in long-term care?

    a. encounter record
    b. registration record
    c. medical history
    d. progress notes

18. Which structured analysis tool most closely resembles a hierarchy chart?

    a. data dictionary
    b. data flow diagram
    c. decomposition diagram
    d. entity-relationship diagram

19. Which of the following is NOT necessary for an authorization for disclosure of patient information to be valid?

    a. It must be addressed to the healthcare provider.
    b. It must state that the authorization may be revoked by the patient or his or her legal representative.
    c. It must be signed by the patient or his or her legal representative.
    d. It must be dated within the past year.

20. Which of the following is an advantage of the case-control study design?

    a. The design makes case-control studies less likely to be influenced by bias than cohort studies.
    b. It is easy to select an appropriate control group for a case-control study.
    c. It is easy to validate the information obtained during a case-control study.
    d. The design results in studies that require fewer subjects than other types of studies.

21. Which of the following is a disadvantage of the prevalence study design?

    a. It is expensive.
    b. It is ineffective for the study of rare diseases.
    c. It rarely leads to secondary research.
    d. It takes a long time to produce observable results.

22. In which numbering system(s) does a patient retain the same number for each of his or her encounters?

    a. serial-unit numbering
    b. serial numbering
    c. unit numbering
    d. all of the above

23. A piece of computer equipment costs $2000. It will be obsolete in five years, at which time it will need to be replaced. If the straight-line method for calculating depreciation is used, what will be the value of the equipment after three years?

    a. $800
    b. $1000
    c. $1200
    d. $2000

24. Which coding system is used most often by AIDS registries?

    a. SNOMED
    b. HCPCS
    c. DSM-5
    d. ICD-9-CM

25. Which of the following scenarios illustrates ascertainment bias?

    a. An interviewer tends to modify his or her style of questioning based on the answers given at the beginning of an interview.
    b. A study is largely based on interviews, and the subjects tend to exaggerate the severity of their ailments.
    c. The subjects of a new research study have received a disproportionate amount of health treatment in the past.
    d. Two pathologists offer conflicting diagnoses when presented with the same set of specimens.

26. In the standard six-digit identification number 12-44-09, the numbers 1 and 2 are known as the

    a. primary digits.
    b. secondary digits.
    c. tertiary digits.
    d. terminal digits.

27. In which of the following situations would the burden of proof shift to the defendant in a malpractice suit?

    a. A patient under general anesthesia remains in a coma for several weeks.
    b. A patient finds that a surgical tool has been inadvertently left in her body.
    c. A patient does not recover full range of motion after rotator cuff surgery.
    d. A patient experiences nausea after taking a prescribed medication.

28. Which of the following coding systems is used in skilled nursing facilities?

    a. ICD-9-CM, vol. 3
    b. HCPCS/CPT
    c. HCFA I 500 billing form
    d. UB-92 billing form

29. The _____ of data is the degree to which it has appropriate specificity.

    a. granularity
    b. relevancy
    c. accuracy
    d. accessibility

30. A healthcare facility determines that it takes 12 minutes to code each inpatient record. A full-time coder works 150 hours every month, and the facility discharges about 3000 inpatients each month. How many coders must be employed by the healthcare facility to keep up with the facility's coding demands?

    a. 2
    b. 4
    c. 6
    d. 8

31. A healthcare facility has $500,000 of current assets and $200,000 of current liabilities. What is the current ratio of the healthcare facility?

    a. 1.8
    b. 2.5
    c. 4.2
    d. 5.2

32. During the month of May, a 500-bed facility had 400 deaths, 2000 other discharges, and 345 comorbidities. What was the comorbidity rate for the month? Round your answer to the nearest tenth of a percent.

    a. 40.0%
    b. 20.8%
    c. 17.3%
    d. 14.4%

33. Which of the following is an advantage of microfilm jackets for micrographics?

    a. The records for several different patients are stored on the same film.
    b. They are a relatively inexpensive option for micrographics.
    c. Jackets are all the same color.
    d. Unit records are created automatically.

34. Which of the following is an example of a keyed entry device?

    a. mark-sense reader
    b. optical scanner
    c. bar code reader
    d. light pen

35. Which of the following statements about HMOs is true?

    a. Insurance providers volunteer to participate in plans.
    b. Subscribers do not make payments unless they utilize healthcare services.
    c. The HMO has an implicit obligation to provide healthcare services.
    d. The financial risk associated with a plan is assumed by the subscriber.

36. An organization conducts a survey about alcohol consumption with the members of a community. Questionnaires accompanied by self-addressed stamped envelopes are mailed to local residents. The results of the survey indicate that the area has a below average rate of alcoholism. What is the most likely reason for these results?

    a. diagnosis bias
    b. nonresponse bias
    c. prevarication bias
    d. survival bias

37. If a test produces 200 true positives, 50 false negatives, 175 true negatives, and 40 false positives, what is the specificity of the test? Round your answer to the nearest percentage point.

    a. 27%
    b. 57%
    c. 81%
    d. 91%

38. A set of data has a mean of –5 and a standard deviation of 2. What is the coefficient of variation for this data set?

    a. –40%
    b. 25%
    c. 40%
    d. 250%

39. A healthcare administrator is responsible for creating staffing budgets. It is estimated that the information desk receives 8000 queries annually. A full-time staff member can handle about 20 queries per day. The employees at the facility typically use nine vacation days and take seven sick days during the year, and there are eleven holidays as well. If the productivity adjustment is taken into account, how many full-time employees should the healthcare administrator allow for in the budget? Round your answer to the nearest tenth.

    a. 1.1
    b. 1.3
    c. 1.7
    d. 2.5

40. Which of the following is an advantage of the decentralized record management system?

    a. The supply costs of storage equipment are decreased.
    b. The format of the files can be more flexible.
    c. It is easier to maintain strict record control.
    d. Training staff responsible for file management is easier.

41. Which piece of legislation established the National Practitioner Data Bank?

    a. the Tax Equity and Fiscal Responsibility Act
    b. the Health Care Quality Improvement Act
    c. the Health Insurance Portability and Accountability Act
    d. the Nursing Home Reform Act

42. Which of the following is an indirect cost of a data system?

a. photocopy supply costs
b. outside service costs
c. interest costs
d. labor costs

43. In which site of care are patient records LEAST likely to contain nursing notes?

a. behavioral healthcare
b. hospice care
c. acute care
d. ambulatory care

44. Which organization is responsible for the level 2 national codes in the HCFA Common Procedure Coding System?

a. the American Medical Association
b. the Health Care Financing Administration
c. local fiscal intermediaries
d. the American Hospital Association

45. Which of the following is a disadvantage of prospective study?

a. Prospective study is expensive.
b. Prospective study only estimates relative risk.
c. Prospective study is subject to recall bias.
d. Prospective study cannot determine whether the symptom preceded the disease.

46. Who may sign the form to authorize the release of confidential information for a minor whose parent is also a minor?

a. the attending physician
b. the patient
c. the parent
d. all of the above

47. During the month of January, a 400-bed healthcare facility had 450 deaths, 2500 other discharges, and 11,000 inpatient service days. What was the inpatient bed occupancy rate for January? Round your answer to the nearest percentage point.

a. 28%
b. 44%
c. 89%
d. 94%

48. Which of the following is a characteristic of the straight numeric filing system?

a. Work is distributed throughout the hundred sections.
b. Records that are not being used are pulled from one area.
c. Every file grows evenly in the hundred sections.
d. Numbers are divided into groups of two.

49. Which piece of legislation created a program for detecting fraudulent health plans?

    a. the Health Insurance Portability and Accountability Act of 1996

    b. the Nursing Home Reform Act of 1987

    c. the Patient Self-Determination Act of 1990

    d. the Consolidated Omnibus Budget Reconciliation Act of 1985

50. If a test produces 400 true positives, 350 true negatives, 50 false positives, and 20 false negatives, what is the sensitivity of the test? Round your answer to the nearest percentage point.

    a. 88%

    b. 90%

    c. 92%

    d. 95%

Answer Key and Explanations

1. A: The Atlas Severity of Illness System presents ordinal data. Ordinal data is organized by rank according to an established set of criteria. The Atlas Severity of Illness System uses a scale from zero to four. Zero indicates no risk of vital organ failure, while four indicates the presence of vital organ failure. Interviews or questionnaires conducted or administered by healthcare facilities often involve collecting ordinal data. Nominal data is the arbitrary assignment of numbers to the representatives of particular categories. For instance, in a nominal system, women might be represented as zero and men as one. Continuous data has no boundary, and a number will have meaning regardless of its value. Temperature and blood pressure are common examples of continuous data. Discrete data is in the form of whole numbers, has some reasonable limitations, and is meaningful. Examples of discrete data include the number of children in a family or the number of milligrams of medication a patient takes per day.

2. D: In the staff model, all of the providers work in the same facility. HMOs that use this model employ a comprehensive set of service providers, all of whom work in the same location. In the group model, the HMO makes arrangements for the provision of services with hospitals and group practices. In an independent practice association, the group of healthcare providers is a legal entity that is separate from the HMO. The group of service providers, known as an IPA, forms working relationships with other practitioners when necessary. In the network type, the HMO makes agreements with scattered service providers, who may or may not serve the subscribers to the HMO exclusively.

3. D: Reasons are not a component of a PERT network. The acronym PERT stands for Program Evaluation Review Technique. This methodology was developed to help administrators sequence complex processes. The three components of a PERT network are goals, events, and activities. The goal is the basic intention of the network. The events in the network are specific activities or groups of activities that will contribute to the achievement of the goal. Activities are the tasks that must be performed in order to move from one event to the other.

4. C: One characteristic of the terminal digit filing system is that each number is divided into pairs of digits. Specifically, each number is divided into three sets of digits. An example is 11-45-87. Social Security numbers use a terminal digit filing system. In the terminal digit filing system, numbers are read from right to left for the purposes of filing, but from left to right for the purposes of identification. Typically, the training period for a terminal digit filing system is longer than the training period required for a straight numeric system. Also, inactive records are purged evenly from the hundred sections of the file, and are not drawn from the same area. In a terminal digit filing system, the file tends to grow at the same pace throughout the hundred sections. This avoids the need for backshifting.

5. C: The case mix index for this period is 1.3. The case mix index is calculated by dividing the total value of service by the total number of cases. In this case, then, the calculation is as follows: 179 ÷ 140 = 1.3. Determining the case mix index enables a healthcare facility to identify how well resources are being used to treat particular ailments.

6. A: The nosocomial infection rate for the facility was 1.2%. This rate is calculated by dividing the number of nosocomial infections by the total number of discharges (including deaths), and then multiplying by 100. So, for this problem, the nosocomial infection rate would be calculated as follows: (35/3000) × 100 = 1.2%.

7. B: The ICD-9-CM coding instrument is generally recommended for principal diagnosis upon admittance to inpatient treatment. The International Classification of Diseases, 9th Edition, Clinical Modification (commonly known as the ICD-9-CM) is used to make the determination that will inform the patient's treatment following admission. The Systematized Nomenclature of Diseases and Operations (SNOMED) makes it possible for distant healthcare facilities to compare the treatment protocols and patient responses for common conditions. The Health Care Financing Administration Common Procedure Coding System (HCPCS) is used on the billing documents for inpatient, ambulatory, and surgical treatment. The Diagnostic and Statistical Manual of Mental Disorders (DSM-5) is the primary coding system for mental conditions.

8. B: In an automated record tracking system, requests are not prioritized manually. On the contrary, automated record tracking systems use a sophisticated software program to prioritize requests. This drastically accelerates the process of handling inquiries. The other answer choices are characteristics of automated record tracking systems. These systems alert staff members of returned records after the staff member returns to his or her workstation. It is possible to configure these systems to keep track of multiple file room locations, and these systems are updated in real time. With these systems, it is possible to request individual records or groups of records instantaneously. Barcode technology can be integrated with these systems, as can keyboard data entry.

9. B: The weighted average length of stay for April is 3.7 days. Weighted average length of stay is a good way to assess the average length of stay per patient. It is a more detailed metric than a simple average of the lengths of stay in each department. Weighted average length of stay is calculated by adding up the products of the number of patients and the average length of stay within each department, and then dividing this sum by the total number of patients. So, in this case, the weighted average length of stay would be calculated as follows: $(25 \times 3 + 50 \times 4) \div (25 + 50) = (75 + 200) \div 75 = 3.7$.

10. B: A balance sheet provides a snapshot of a company's financial position at a specific time. This document, which is also known as the statement of financial position, summarizes the assets, liabilities, and equity of an organization. An income statement reports the revenues, expenses, and net income (or loss) for a given period. The statement of owner's equity, also known as the retained earnings statement, reports changes in an owner's capital account over a given period. A statement of cash flows summarizes all of the cash receipts and payments during an accounting period.

11. A: The dimension of performance addressed by this study is efficacy. When used to describe the provision of health services, efficacy is the extent to which an activity achieves its intended outcome. The study in this question, then, is measuring the efficacy of the guidelines provided by the American Dental Association. It is important for a medical service authority to understand how often and how exactly its recommendations are followed. The appropriateness of an activity is the extent to which it applies to the clinical needs of the patient. Continuity is the extent to which multiple healthcare providers are able to coordinate and maintain consistent therapy for patients over a long duration. Finally, the efficiency of healthcare activity is the extent to which desired outcomes are achieved with a minimum use of resources.

12. B: The American Hospital Association maintains the Central Office on ICD-9-CM. This organization is also responsible for publishing Coding Clinic and approving official coding guidelines. The National Center for Health Statistics is responsible for maintaining the classification system for diseases. The American Health Information Management Association provides certification to health coders and administrates coding education programs. AHIMA also sponsors

the Society for Clinical Coding and the Council on Coding and Classification. The Health Care Financing Administration is responsible for the classification of medical procedures.

13. A: Blood pressure measurements are an example of continuous data. Continuous data has the potential to remain meaningful through an infinite number of values. Weight and cost are two classic examples of continuous data, since, theoretically, there is no upper limit to either. Discrete data, on the other hand, consists of meaningful whole numbers. There is an upper limit, even though this limit may be unknown. An example of discrete data would be the number of patients admitted by a healthcare facility during a particular interval. Nominal data is simply the set of numbers assigned to different categories. In nominal data sets, the exact values assigned are arbitrary. For instance, there is no real reason why females must be coded as 0 and males coded as 1, and not vice versa. Ordinal data indicates the position or rank of the data within a value set. A common example of ordinal data is the five-point self-assessment scale that is used by patients to describe their current health status.

14. D: The resources-based relative value system is the Medicare reimbursement methodology used in physician offices and clinics. In this system, services are compared to a standard value of 1.0. In other words, a service that is two-and-a-half times as significant as the standard service will receive a value of 2.5. The prospective payment system per diem is used in skilled nursing facilities. The ambulatory surgery center groups reimbursement system is used in freestanding ambulatory surgery centers. The prospective payment system based on diagnosis-related groups is used by hospital inpatient facilities.

15. B: The mode of the data set is 6. In statistics, the mode of a data set is the value that appears most often. In the given data set, the only value that appears more than once is 6. It is also important to know how to calculate the mean and median of a data set. The mean, also known as the average, is calculated by adding the values together and dividing by the number of values in the set. For this set, the mean would be calculated as follows: $(1 + 4 + 6 + 6 + 8 + 9 + 12 + 15 + 18) / 9 = 8.78$. The median of a data set is the value that falls in the middle when the values are placed in order from least to greatest. For this data set, the median is 8.

16. D: The total value of service for July was 56. Total value of service is calculated by multiplying the case mix value by the number of cases recorded during the period. So, in this scenario, the total value of service would be calculated as follows: $1.4 \times 40 = 56$.

17. A: Of the given data items, an encounter record is least likely to appear on the clinical forms of a patient in long-term care. Indeed, it is quite possible that this record will never appear on clinical forms for long-term care patients. The encounter record is a typical component of ambulatory care record keeping, and is used during the billing process. It would include the basic diagnosis and treatment protocol. Registration records, medical history, and progress notes will almost always be a part of the clinical forms for a patient in long-term care. The registration record typically includes the basic diagnosis, as well as the allergies and sensitivities of the patient. This record should be legible, and the use of symbols and abbreviations should be avoided. The medical history is typically provided by the patient, and should include the chief complaint, symptoms, history of illness, family history, and a basic review of systems. Progress notes, finally, provide a record of the patient's response to treatment.

18. C: Decomposition diagrams closely resemble a hierarchy chart. A decomposition diagram subdivides a complex problem into a set of smaller problems. The relationships between complex problems and their constituent elements are represented in a manner similar to a family tree. A data dictionary is a technique for modeling data in which all of the elements and structures are

compiled. A data flow diagram is a depiction of the patterns of movement for data within a system. This could be the physical or procedural flow. An entity-relationship diagram is a technique for modeling data in which the sequential design of the database schema is represented.

19. D: A date within the past year is not necessary for an authorization for disclosure of patient information to be valid. Instead, in most jurisdictions, the form must be dated within the last six months, and in some places within an even shorter time frame. It is necessary, however, for an authorization for disclosure of patient information to be addressed to the healthcare provider. It must state that the authorization may be revoked by the patient or his or her legal representative. This authorization must also be signed by the patient or his or her legal representative. Moreover, the authorization must be in writing, and must give the patient's full name, address, and date of birth. It must identify the party authorized to receive the information, as well as the information that is to be released. It must explain the reason for the disclosure, and must name a date upon which the authorization will expire, assuming it has not already been revoked. Finally, it must state that the authorization may be revoked by the patient or by his or her legal representative.

20. D: One advantage of the case-control design is that studies that employ this design require fewer subjects than studies that employ other designs. Some other advantages of studies that use this design are that they are relatively inexpensive, they allow for the use of already existing records, and they pose only a slight risk to subjects. Case-control studies also produce results faster than prospective or cohort studies. However, case-control studies can be easily influenced by recall bias, and it can be very difficult to select an appropriate control group for such a study. Also, validating the information acquired during a case-control study can be difficult.

21. B: One disadvantage of the prevalence study design is that it is ineffective for the study of rare diseases. The prevalence study design measures the distribution of symptoms or diseases in different populations at a particular moment. This case study design is very useful for generating hypotheses that can be tested through subsequent research. It is typically inexpensive, and tends to produce observable results quickly. However, prevalence studies are unable to suggest causal relationships, and their use is limited to those members of the population who are still alive to be tested.

22. C: In a unit numbering system, the patient retains the same number for each of his or her encounters. Each patient's record is filed according to his or her unit number. In both the serial and serial-unit numbering systems, a patient receives a new number for each encounter. Many healthcare facilities find that adopting a unit numbering system eliminates a great deal of work, and also prevents file folders from being spread out over disparate locations.

23. A: If the straight-line method for calculating depreciation is used, the value of the equipment after three years will be $800. In the straight-line method of depreciation, objects are considered to decline in value by a regular amount every year until they are obsolete or need to be replaced. In this case, then, the computer equipment's annual amount of depreciation is calculated by dividing its original price by the number of years it will be in service: $2000 ÷ 5 = $400. The equipment will depreciate at a rate of $400 per year, so the amount of depreciation after three years can be calculated as follows: $400 × 3 = $1200. This is subtracted from the original price to yield the value of the equipment after three years: $2000 – $1200 = $800.

24. D: The ICD-9-CM coding system is used most often by AIDS registries. It is extremely important for health officials to monitor the spread of AIDS and patterns of AIDS incidences. The International Classification of Diseases, 9th Edition, Clinical Modification (ICD-9-CM) is the preferred coding system for admission. The Systematized Nomenclature of Diseases and Operations (SNOMED)

- 94 -

enables the treatment protocols for common ailments at disparate facilities to be compared. The Health Care Financing Administration Common Procedure Coding System (HCPCS) is commonly used by the billing departments of healthcare facilities. The Diagnostic and Statistical Manual of Mental Disorders (DSM-5) is the primary coding system and the repository of diagnostic criteria for mental conditions.

25. C: A scenario in which the subjects of a new research study receive a disproportionate amount of health treatment prior to the study is an example of ascertainment bias. Ascertainment bias is the tendency of researchers to select research subjects who receive a greater amount of medical treatment more often. This often occurs when the volunteer population of a research study is likely to be composed of people with a special interest in physical fitness or nutrition. When the interviewer modifies his or her style of questioning based on the answers given early in the interview, it is known as interviewer bias. Interviewer bias can be resolved by standardizing the question sequence. When subjects are apt to exaggerate the severity of their ailments, it is known as prevarication bias. Prevarication bias is especially common in situations where research subjects have some incentive to manifest a particular medical condition, such as when they are receiving disability compensation. When two pathologists offer conflicting diagnoses of the same specimens, it is known as diagnosis bias. Diagnosis bias can often be resolved by preventing the pathologists from knowing the provenance of the specimens.

26. C: In the standard six-digit identification number 12-44-09, the numbers 1 and 2 are known as the tertiary digits. The middle digits are known as the secondary digits, and the digits on the right are called the primary or terminal digits. In a terminal digit filing system, numbers are read from right to left during filing operations, but are read from left to right for identification purposes.

27. B: If a patient discovers that a surgical tool has been inadvertently left in her body, the burden of proof in the malpractice suit shifts to the defendant. This shift is based on the legal concept of res ipsa loquitur, or "a situation that speaks for itself." In this case, it is obvious that the nature of the injury indicates negligence, and that the plaintiff could have had no role in her injury. In order for the burden of proof to shift to the defendant in a malpractice suit, it must be clear that the injury would not have occurred without negligence, that the defendant was totally in control of the process that caused the injury, and that the plaintiff made no contribution to the injury. Of the answer choices, only B meets all of these criteria.

28. D: The UB-92 billing form is the coding system used in skilled nursing facilities. These facilities also use the first two volumes of the ICD-9-CM coding system. The ICD-9-CM, vol. 3 is used in hospital inpatient and outpatient facilities, as well as in hospital-based ambulatory surgery centers. It is often used in freestanding ambulatory surgery centers. The HCPCS/CPT billing form is required for Medicare in hospital outpatient and hospital-based ambulatory surgery centers. It is also used in freestanding ambulatory surgery centers and physician offices and clinics. The HCFA I 500 billing form is used in freestanding ambulatory surgery centers and physician offices and clinics.

29. A: The granularity of data is the degree to which it has appropriate specificity. The relevancy of data is the extent to which it applies to the process or function for which it was collected. The accuracy of data is its correctness. The accessibility of data is the ease and legality with which it may be collected.

30. B: The healthcare facility needs four coders. The number of coders is calculated by dividing the product of the coding time required per record and the number of discharges and/or visits for the period by the number of paid hours worked per coder during the time period: "coding time per record × # of discharges and/or visits per period" /"# of paid hours worked per coder for the time

- 95 -

period". It is important to note that 12 minutes is 1/5, or 0.2, of an hour. The number of coders required is determined in the following manner: $(0.2 \times 3000)/150 = 4$.

31. B: The current ratio of the healthcare facility is 2.5. Current ratio, which is one of the most common liquidity ratios used in finance, is simply a comparison of current assets and current liabilities. In this case, it is calculated in the following way: $500,000/200,000 = 2.5$. Values for current assets and current liabilities would be found on a balance sheet. The general purpose of the current ratio is to indicate whether a business has enough cash and/or liquid assets to cover its short-term obligations.

32. D: The comorbidity rate for this facility during the month of May was 14.4%. Comorbidity refers to a condition that a patient has upon being admitted, is different from the condition for which a patient is being admitted, and increases a patient's stay by at least a day three-quarters of the time. Comorbidity rate is calculated by dividing the total number of comorbidities by the total number of discharges (including deaths), and then multiplying the quotient by 100. So, in this scenario, the comorbidity rate would be calculated as follows: $[345 \div (400 + 2000)] \times 100 = [345 \div 2400] \times 100 = 0.14375 \times 100 = 14.375\%$, or 14.4%.

33. D: One advantage of microfilm jackets for micrographics is that unit records are created automatically. In a microfilm jacket system, individual files are represented on pieces of film cut out of a continuous roll. These pieces of film are placed in groups of up to seventy in 4×6 containers. This is the most expensive micrographics option, but it allows patient records to be stored individually, which is useful when records need to be exported. The jackets may be the same color, but most facilities find it helpful to use a color coding system for microfilm jackets.

34. D: A light pen is a keyed entry device. A keyed entry device uses a graphical user interface similar to a Windows desktop. A light pen is a special instrument that is applied directly to the display screen to enter information. Mark-sense readers, optical scanners, and bar code readers are all examples of scanned entry devices. A scanned entry device uses a piece of sensory equipment to read information and transport it to its memory system. In a mark-sense reader system, employees use a pencil to darken circles on a form, which is then fed into a machine and entered into memory. A mark-sense reader functions much like a standardized multiple choice test. An optical scanner transmits the image of a paper document into a computer's memory. A bar code reader obtains information from a series of varying black vertical stripes on the document. Bar codes are considered to be extremely accurate, though they may be time-consuming to create.

35. A: In an HMO, insurance providers volunteer to participate in the plan. This is one of the essential characteristics of the health maintenance organization model for health insurance provision. Moreover, subscriber participation in HMOs is voluntary. The other answer choices are incorrect statements about HMOs. Subscribers are required to make a fixed minimum payment monthly, regardless of whether they use services. The HMO's obligation to provide healthcare service is not implicit; it is explicitly outlined in the contract agreed upon by the subscriber and the provider. Finally, in the HMO model, the financial risk is assumed by the HMO, not the subscriber.

36. B: The most likely reason for the results in this scenario is nonresponse bias. Nonresponse bias occurs when it is probable that survey respondents will have significantly different characteristics than survey non-respondents. In this scenario, it seems likely that cultural pressures would encourage people to underreport their alcohol consumption. Heavy drinkers might avoid reporting any consumption at all. Diagnosis bias, on the other hand, occurs when there is disagreement among professionals about the meaning of specimens collected during a research study. A prevarication bias exists when survey respondents embellish their answers, either by exaggerating

their characteristics or providing obfuscating details. Survival bias occurs when the results of a study are influenced by the fact that the members of a population who are still alive are more likely to share certain characteristics. For instance, a study of 80-year-old lifelong smokers might produce a smaller than expected incidence of cancer, for the simple reason that other lifelong smokers would have died of the disease by this age.

37. C: If a test produces 200 true positives, 50 false negatives, 175 true negatives, and 40 false positives, the specificity of the test is 81%. The specificity of a test is the percentage of all true non-cases that are identified. In other words, specificity is a measure of how successful a test is at identifying members of a population who do not have a condition. Specificity is calculated by dividing the number of true negatives by the total number of non-cases (the sum of true negatives and false positives). In this scenario, specificity is calculated as follows: 175 / (175 + 40) = 175 / 215 = 81%.

38. C: The coefficient of variation for this data set is 40%. The coefficient of variation is calculated so that the standard deviations of different samples or groups may be compared. It is determined by dividing the standard deviation by the absolute value (distance from zero) of the mean, and then multiplying by 100. So, for this problem, the calculation would be done as follows: "CV=" $s/|\bar{x}|$ ×100=2/5×100=40%. Remember that the absolute value of –5 is 5. The coefficient of variation will always be a positive value.

39. C: The healthcare administrator will need to allot funds for 1.7 full-time employees in the budget. This is a complex calculation, particularly when the productivity adjustment is made. To begin with, it is necessary to calculate the number of full-time employees that would be required if employees worked every day. This is done by first multiplying the number of queries an employee can handle by the number of days in a work week and the number of weeks in a year: 20 × 5 × 52 = 5200. This is the total number of queries that a full-time employee could handle in a year if he or she worked every day. For this ideal scenario, the number of required employees can be calculated by dividing the total number of requests by the number of requests each employee can handle: 8000 ÷ 5200 = 1.5. However, it is noted in the question that employees do not actually work every day. Full-time employees miss an average of 27 days each, which can be multiplied by the number of hours in a day to yield the total number of non-productive hours: 27 × 8 = 216. The amount of actual productive time for each employee can then be calculated by subtracting these non-productive hours from the ideal productive time, which is 2080 (this is calculated by multiplying the number of hours in a work day by the number of days in a work week by the number of weeks in a year). This calculation is done as follows: 2080 – 216 = 1864. The productivity rate is calculated by dividing the amount of real productive time by the total possible amount of productive time: 1864 ÷ 2080 = .896 = 90%. The actual number of full-time employees that need to be included in the budget can then be calculated by dividing the number of full-time employees required in the ideal productivity calculation by the productivity rate adjustment: 1.5/90% = 1.7 full-time employees.

40. B: One advantage of the decentralized record management system is that the format of files can be more flexible. This allows healthcare facilities to adapt the system to the unique needs of the healthcare provider or patients. In a decentralized system, filing units are spread throughout the facility. This arrangement is common when the institution contains a number of specialty departments. Unfortunately, the supply costs associated with storage equipment for a decentralized record management system are significantly higher, and it is harder to maintain strict record control. Finally, it is more difficult to train staff to use a decentralized filing system.

41. B: The Health Care Quality Improvement Act established the National Practitioner Data Bank in 1986. The National Practitioner Data Bank assembles and disseminates information about incompetent or malpracticing healthcare service providers. The Health Insurance Portability and Accountability Act improved the quality of health insurance and created a program for detecting fraud and abuse in health plans. The Tax Equity and Fiscal Responsibility Act (TEFRA) made significant changes to the Medicare reimbursement structure. The Nursing Home Reform Act established minimum staffing requirements for long-term care facilities.

42. C: Interest is an indirect cost of a data system. When evaluating the costs and benefits of a proposed data system, it is important to consider both the direct and indirect costs. For instance, the direct costs are those that may be easily defined. Every data system will involve labor and its associated costs. Many systems will necessarily incur photocopy supply costs and microfilm costs. It is inevitable that outside service will be required as well. It is rarely possible, though, to precisely estimate the amount of interest that will be owed because of billing delays, especially when the facility's system is based on paper.

43. D: Patient records related to ambulatory care are the least likely to contain nursing notes. Nursing notes outline the patient's condition and treatment protocol in specific terms. A set of nursing notes typically includes an admission note and a summary of all nursing interventions, including a description of the patient's response. The concluding document in a series of nursing notes will be the discharge record. Because nursing notes pertain explicitly to inpatient treatment, they are rarely created for ambulatory patients.

44. B: The Health Care Financing Administration is responsible for the level 2 national codes in the HCFA Common Procedure Coding System (HCPCS). The HCPCS is a common coding system for health care. It is divided into three levels. Level 1 of the HCPCS, Current Procedural Terminology, is overseen by the American Medical Association. This portion of the coding system contains six sections: evaluation and management, anesthesiology, surgery, radiology, pathology, and medicine. Level 3, the set of local codes, is maintained by local fiscal intermediaries and carriers.

45. A: One disadvantage of prospective study is that it is very expensive. Some other disadvantages of this type of system are that it takes a long time to produce results, and it can be easily influenced by unpredictable changes in the environment or the behavior patterns of participants. Also, prospective study is not good at obtaining information about rare diseases. However, prospective study is able to determine relative risk exactly, and it is notably devoid of recall bias. Moreover, a prospective study is usually able to identify whether the symptom preceded the disease.

46. C: The parent of a minor may sign the form to authorize the release of confidential information, even when the parent is also a minor. This is a special scenario, in which authorization cannot simply be given by the patient or the patient's legal representative. When a patient is a minor, authorization may always be given by his or her parent or legal guardian. When a patient has been deemed to be legally incompetent, authorization may be given by his or her legally appointed guardian. When a patient is an emancipated minor, authorization may be given by the patient.

47. C: The inpatient bed occupancy rate for the month of January was about 89%. This census statistic is also called the occupancy rate, occupancy percentage, or percentage of occupancy. The inpatient bed occupancy rate is calculated by dividing the number of inpatient service days by the product of the number of beds and the number of days in the month, and then multiplying by 100. So, for this question, inpatient bed occupancy rate is calculated as follows: $[11,000 \div (400 \times 31)] \times 100 = [11,000 \div 12,400] \times 100 = 0.887 \times 100 = 88.7\%$.

48. B: One characteristic of the straight numeric filing system is that records not currently being used are pulled from one area. A straight numeric filing system is a simple manner for organizing files: each file is assigned a number, and new files receive the next number in the sequence (e.g., 14556, 14557, 14558...). In a straight numeric filing system, work is not distributed evenly, but is instead concentrated in the highest numbers, since these are the most recent additions and therefore the most likely to be active. Inactive records are pulled from one general area, unlike in a terminal digit filing system, in which inactive records are purged evenly throughout the hundred sections. Similarly, the files in a straight numeric filing system grow at the end of the number sequence, and so it is necessary to backshift files in order to create space. Finally, in a straight numeric filing system numbers are represented as a whole, whereas in the terminal digit filing system they are divided into pairs of digits.

49. A: The Health Insurance Portability and Accountability Act created a program for detecting fraudulent health plans. This act, passed in 1996 and implemented in 1998, generally improved the quality, access, and affordability of health insurance. The Nursing Home Reform Act, passed in 1987 and made effective in 1990, established minimum staffing requirements for long-term care facilities. The Patient Self-Determination Act, passed in 1990, mandated a wider dissemination of information to patients about their health options and rights. The Consolidated Omnibus Budget Reconciliation Act of 1985, commonly known as COBRA, established standards for the transfer and discharge of Medicaid and Medicare recipients.

50. D: If a test produces 400 true positives, 350 true negatives, 50 false positives, and 20 false negatives, the sensitivity of the test is 95%. The sensitivity of a test is calculated by dividing the number of true positives by the number of total positives (the sum of true positives and false negatives). In this scenario, then, sensitivity is calculated as follows: 400 / (400 + 20) = 400 / 420 = 95.2%. The sensitivity of a test is the percentage of all true cases correctly identified by the test.

How to Overcome Test Anxiety

Just the thought of taking a test is enough to make most people a little nervous. A test is an important event that can have a long-term impact on your future, so it's important to take it seriously and it's natural to feel anxious about performing well. But just because anxiety is normal, that doesn't mean that it's helpful in test taking, or that you should simply accept it as part of your life. Anxiety can have a variety of effects. These effects can be mild, like making you feel slightly nervous, or severe, like blocking your ability to focus or remember even a simple detail.

If you experience test anxiety—whether severe or mild—it's important to know how to beat it. To discover this, first you need to understand what causes test anxiety.

Causes of Test Anxiety

While we often think of anxiety as an uncontrollable emotional state, it can actually be caused by simple, practical things. One of the most common causes of test anxiety is that a person does not feel adequately prepared for their test. This feeling can be the result of many different issues such as poor study habits or lack of organization, but the most common culprit is time management. Starting to study too late, failing to organize your study time to cover all of the material, or being distracted while you study will mean that you're not well prepared for the test. This may lead to cramming the night before, which will cause you to be physically and mentally exhausted for the test. Poor time management also contributes to feelings of stress, fear, and hopelessness as you realize you are not well prepared but don't know what to do about it.

Other times, test anxiety is not related to your preparation for the test but comes from unresolved fear. This may be a past failure on a test, or poor performance on tests in general. It may come from comparing yourself to others who seem to be performing better or from the stress of living up to expectations. Anxiety may be driven by fears of the future—how failure on this test would affect your educational and career goals. These fears are often completely irrational, but they can still negatively impact your test performance.

> **Review Video:** 3 Reasons You Have Test Anxiety
> Visit mometrix.com/academy and enter code: 428468

Elements of Test Anxiety

As mentioned earlier, test anxiety is considered to be an emotional state, but it has physical and mental components as well. Sometimes you may not even realize that you are suffering from test anxiety until you notice the physical symptoms. These can include trembling hands, rapid heartbeat, sweating, nausea, and tense muscles. Extreme anxiety may lead to fainting or vomiting. Obviously, any of these symptoms can have a negative impact on testing. It is important to recognize them as soon as they begin to occur so that you can address the problem before it damages your performance.

> **Review Video: 3 Ways to Tell You Have Test Anxiety**
> Visit mometrix.com/academy and enter code: 927847

The mental components of test anxiety include trouble focusing and inability to remember learned information. During a test, your mind is on high alert, which can help you recall information and stay focused for an extended period of time. However, anxiety interferes with your mind's natural processes, causing you to blank out, even on the questions you know well. The strain of testing during anxiety makes it difficult to stay focused, especially on a test that may take several hours. Extreme anxiety can take a huge mental toll, making it difficult not only to recall test information but even to understand the test questions or pull your thoughts together.

> **Review Video: How Test Anxiety Affects Memory**
> Visit mometrix.com/academy and enter code: 609003

Effects of Test Anxiety

Test anxiety is like a disease—if left untreated, it will get progressively worse. Anxiety leads to poor performance, and this reinforces the feelings of fear and failure, which in turn lead to poor performances on subsequent tests. It can grow from a mild nervousness to a crippling condition. If allowed to progress, test anxiety can have a big impact on your schooling, and consequently on your future.

Test anxiety can spread to other parts of your life. Anxiety on tests can become anxiety in any stressful situation, and blanking on a test can turn into panicking in a job situation. But fortunately, you don't have to let anxiety rule your testing and determine your grades. There are a number of relatively simple steps you can take to move past anxiety and function normally on a test and in the rest of life.

> **Review Video: How Test Anxiety Impacts Your Grades**
> Visit mometrix.com/academy and enter code: 939819

Physical Steps for Beating Test Anxiety

While test anxiety is a serious problem, the good news is that it can be overcome. It doesn't have to control your ability to think and remember information. While it may take time, you can begin taking steps today to beat anxiety.

Just as your first hint that you may be struggling with anxiety comes from the physical symptoms, the first step to treating it is also physical. Rest is crucial for having a clear, strong mind. If you are tired, it is much easier to give in to anxiety. But if you establish good sleep habits, your body and mind will be ready to perform optimally, without the strain of exhaustion. Additionally, sleeping well helps you to retain information better, so you're more likely to recall the answers when you see the test questions.

Getting good sleep means more than going to bed on time. It's important to allow your brain time to relax. Take study breaks from time to time so it doesn't get overworked, and don't study right before bed. Take time to rest your mind before trying to rest your body, or you may find it difficult to fall asleep.

> **Review Video: The Importance of Sleep for Your Brain**
> Visit mometrix.com/academy and enter code: 319338

Along with sleep, other aspects of physical health are important in preparing for a test. Good nutrition is vital for good brain function. Sugary foods and drinks may give a burst of energy but this burst is followed by a crash, both physically and emotionally. Instead, fuel your body with protein and vitamin-rich foods.

Also, drink plenty of water. Dehydration can lead to headaches and exhaustion, especially if your brain is already under stress from the rigors of the test. Particularly if your test is a long one, drink water during the breaks. And if possible, take an energy-boosting snack to eat between sections.

> **Review Video: How Diet Can Affect your Mood**
> Visit mometrix.com/academy and enter code: 624317

Along with sleep and diet, a third important part of physical health is exercise. Maintaining a steady workout schedule is helpful, but even taking 5-minute study breaks to walk can help get your blood pumping faster and clear your head. Exercise also releases endorphins, which contribute to a positive feeling and can help combat test anxiety.

When you nurture your physical health, you are also contributing to your mental health. If your body is healthy, your mind is much more likely to be healthy as well. So take time to rest, nourish your body with healthy food and water, and get moving as much as possible. Taking these physical steps will make you stronger and more able to take the mental steps necessary to overcome test anxiety.

> **Review Video: How to Stay Healthy and Prevent Test Anxiety**
> Visit mometrix.com/academy and enter code: 877894

Mental Steps for Beating Test Anxiety

Working on the mental side of test anxiety can be more challenging, but as with the physical side, there are clear steps you can take to overcome it. As mentioned earlier, test anxiety often stems from lack of preparation, so the obvious solution is to prepare for the test. Effective studying may be the most important weapon you have for beating test anxiety, but you can and should employ several other mental tools to combat fear.

First, boost your confidence by reminding yourself of past success—tests or projects that you aced. If you're putting as much effort into preparing for this test as you did for those, there's no reason you should expect to fail here. Work hard to prepare; then trust your preparation.

Second, surround yourself with encouraging people. It can be helpful to find a study group, but be sure that the people you're around will encourage a positive attitude. If you spend time with others who are anxious or cynical, this will only contribute to your own anxiety. Look for others who are motivated to study hard from a desire to succeed, not from a fear of failure.

Third, reward yourself. A test is physically and mentally tiring, even without anxiety, and it can be helpful to have something to look forward to. Plan an activity following the test, regardless of the outcome, such as going to a movie or getting ice cream.

When you are taking the test, if you find yourself beginning to feel anxious, remind yourself that you know the material. Visualize successfully completing the test. Then take a few deep, relaxing breaths and return to it. Work through the questions carefully but with confidence, knowing that you are capable of succeeding.

Developing a healthy mental approach to test taking will also aid in other areas of life. Test anxiety affects more than just the actual test—it can be damaging to your mental health and even contribute to depression. It's important to beat test anxiety before it becomes a problem for more than testing.

> **Review Video: Test Anxiety and Depression**
> Visit mometrix.com/academy and enter code: 904704

Study Strategy

Being prepared for the test is necessary to combat anxiety, but what does being prepared look like? You may study for hours on end and still not feel prepared. What you need is a strategy for test prep. The next few pages outline our recommended steps to help you plan out and conquer the challenge of preparation.

Step 1: Scope Out the Test

Learn everything you can about the format (multiple choice, essay, etc.) and what will be on the test. Gather any study materials, course outlines, or sample exams that may be available. Not only will this help you to prepare, but knowing what to expect can help to alleviate test anxiety.

Step 2: Map Out the Material

Look through the textbook or study guide and make note of how many chapters or sections it has. Then divide these over the time you have. For example, if a book has 15 chapters and you have five days to study, you need to cover three chapters each day. Even better, if you have the time, leave an extra day at the end for overall review after you have gone through the material in depth.

If time is limited, you may need to prioritize the material. Look through it and make note of which sections you think you already have a good grasp on, and which need review. While you are studying, skim quickly through the familiar sections and take more time on the challenging parts. Write out your plan so you don't get lost as you go. Having a written plan also helps you feel more in control of the study, so anxiety is less likely to arise from feeling overwhelmed at the amount to cover. A sample plan may look like this:

- Day 1: Skim chapters 1–4, study chapter 5 (especially pages 31–33)
- Day 2: Study chapters 6–7, skim chapters 8–9
- Day 3: Skim chapter 10, study chapters 11–12 (especially pages 87–90)
- Day 4: Study chapters 13–15
- Day 5: Overall review (focus most on chapters 5, 6, and 12), take practice test

Step 3: Gather Your Tools

Decide what study method works best for you. Do you prefer to highlight in the book as you study and then go back over the highlighted portions? Or do you type out notes of the important information? Or is it helpful to make flashcards that you can carry with you? Assemble the pens, index cards, highlighters, post-it notes, and any other materials you may need so you won't be distracted by getting up to find things while you study.

If you're having a hard time retaining the information or organizing your notes, experiment with different methods. For example, try color-coding by subject with colored pens, highlighters, or post-it notes. If you learn better by hearing, try recording yourself reading your notes so you can listen while in the car, working out, or simply sitting at your desk. Ask a friend to quiz you from your flashcards, or try teaching someone the material to solidify it in your mind.

Step 4: Create Your Environment

It's important to avoid distractions while you study. This includes both the obvious distractions like visitors and the subtle distractions like an uncomfortable chair (or a too-comfortable couch that makes you want to fall asleep). Set up the best study environment possible: good lighting and a comfortable work area. If background music helps you focus, you may want to turn it on, but otherwise keep the room quiet. If you are using a computer to take notes, be sure you don't have any other windows open, especially applications like social media, games, or anything else that could distract you. Silence your phone and turn off notifications. Be sure to keep water close by so you stay hydrated while you study (but avoid unhealthy drinks and snacks).

Also, take into account the best time of day to study. Are you freshest first thing in the morning? Try to set aside some time then to work through the material. Is your mind clearer in the afternoon or evening? Schedule your study session then. Another method is to study at the same time of day that you will take the test, so that your brain gets used to working on the material at that time and will be ready to focus at test time.

Step 5: Study!

Once you have done all the study preparation, it's time to settle into the actual studying. Sit down, take a few moments to settle your mind so you can focus, and begin to follow your study plan. Don't give in to distractions or let yourself procrastinate. This is your time to prepare so you'll be ready to fearlessly approach the test. Make the most of the time and stay focused.

Of course, you don't want to burn out. If you study too long you may find that you're not retaining the information very well. Take regular study breaks. For example, taking five minutes out of every hour to walk briskly, breathing deeply and swinging your arms, can help your mind stay fresh.

As you get to the end of each chapter or section, it's a good idea to do a quick review. Remind yourself of what you learned and work on any difficult parts. When you feel that you've mastered the material, move on to the next part. At the end of your study session, briefly skim through your notes again.

But while review is helpful, cramming last minute is NOT. If at all possible, work ahead so that you won't need to fit all your study into the last day. Cramming overloads your brain with more information than it can process and retain, and your tired mind may struggle to recall even previously learned information when it is overwhelmed with last-minute study. Also, the urgent nature of cramming and the stress placed on your brain contribute to anxiety. You'll be more likely to go to the test feeling unprepared and having trouble thinking clearly.

So don't cram, and don't stay up late before the test, even just to review your notes at a leisurely pace. Your brain needs rest more than it needs to go over the information again. In fact, plan to finish your studies by noon or early afternoon the day before the test. Give your brain the rest of the day to relax or focus on other things, and get a good night's sleep. Then you will be fresh for the test and better able to recall what you've studied.

Step 6: Take a practice test

Many courses offer sample tests, either online or in the study materials. This is an excellent resource to check whether you have mastered the material, as well as to prepare for the test format and environment.

Check the test format ahead of time: the number of questions, the type (multiple choice, free response, etc.), and the time limit. Then create a plan for working through them. For example, if you have 30 minutes to take a 60-question test, your limit is 30 seconds per question. Spend less time on the questions you know well so that you can take more time on the difficult ones.

If you have time to take several practice tests, take the first one open book, with no time limit. Work through the questions at your own pace and make sure you fully understand them. Gradually work up to taking a test under test conditions: sit at a desk with all study materials put away and set a timer. Pace yourself to make sure you finish the test with time to spare and go back to check your answers if you have time.

After each test, check your answers. On the questions you missed, be sure you understand why you missed them. Did you misread the question (tests can use tricky wording)? Did you forget the information? Or was it something you hadn't learned? Go back and study any shaky areas that the practice tests reveal.

Taking these tests not only helps with your grade, but also aids in combating test anxiety. If you're already used to the test conditions, you're less likely to worry about it, and working through tests until you're scoring well gives you a confidence boost. Go through the practice tests until you feel comfortable, and then you can go into the test knowing that you're ready for it.

Test Tips

On test day, you should be confident, knowing that you've prepared well and are ready to answer the questions. But aside from preparation, there are several test day strategies you can employ to maximize your performance.

First, as stated before, get a good night's sleep the night before the test (and for several nights before that, if possible). Go into the test with a fresh, alert mind rather than staying up late to study.

Try not to change too much about your normal routine on the day of the test. It's important to eat a nutritious breakfast, but if you normally don't eat breakfast at all, consider eating just a protein bar. If you're a coffee drinker, go ahead and have your normal coffee. Just make sure you time it so that the caffeine doesn't wear off right in the middle of your test. Avoid sugary beverages, and drink enough water to stay hydrated but not so much that you need a restroom break 10 minutes into the test. If your test isn't first thing in the morning, consider going for a walk or doing a light workout before the test to get your blood flowing.

Allow yourself enough time to get ready, and leave for the test with plenty of time to spare so you won't have the anxiety of scrambling to arrive in time. Another reason to be early is to select a good seat. It's helpful to sit away from doors and windows, which can be distracting. Find a good seat, get out your supplies, and settle your mind before the test begins.

When the test begins, start by going over the instructions carefully, even if you already know what to expect. Make sure you avoid any careless mistakes by following the directions.

Then begin working through the questions, pacing yourself as you've practiced. If you're not sure on an answer, don't spend too much time on it, and don't let it shake your confidence. Either skip it and come back later, or eliminate as many wrong answers as possible and guess among the remaining ones. Don't dwell on these questions as you continue—put them out of your mind and focus on what lies ahead.

Be sure to read all of the answer choices, even if you're sure the first one is the right answer. Sometimes you'll find a better one if you keep reading. But don't second-guess yourself if you do immediately know the answer. Your gut instinct is usually right. Don't let test anxiety rob you of the information you know.

If you have time at the end of the test (and if the test format allows), go back and review your answers. Be cautious about changing any, since your first instinct tends to be correct, but make sure you didn't misread any of the questions or accidentally mark the wrong answer choice. Look over any you skipped and make an educated guess.

At the end, leave the test feeling confident. You've done your best, so don't waste time worrying about your performance or wishing you could change anything. Instead, celebrate the successful completion of this test. And finally, use this test to learn how to deal with anxiety even better next time.

> **Review Video:** 5 Tips to Beat Test Anxiety
> Visit mometrix.com/academy and enter code: 570656

Important Qualification

Not all anxiety is created equal. If your test anxiety is causing major issues in your life beyond the classroom or testing center, or if you are experiencing troubling physical symptoms related to your anxiety, it may be a sign of a serious physiological or psychological condition. If this sounds like your situation, we strongly encourage you to seek professional help.

Thank You

We at Mometrix would like to extend our heartfelt thanks to you, our friend and patron, for allowing us to play a part in your journey. It is a privilege to serve people from all walks of life who are unified in their commitment to building the best future they can for themselves.

The preparation you devote to these important testing milestones may be the most valuable educational opportunity you have for making a real difference in your life. We encourage you to put your heart into it—that feeling of succeeding, overcoming, and yes, conquering will be well worth the hours you've invested.

We want to hear your story, your struggles and your successes, and if you see any opportunities for us to improve our materials so we can help others even more effectively in the future, please share that with us as well. **The team at Mometrix would be absolutely thrilled to hear from you!** So please, send us an email (support@mometrix.com) and let's stay in touch.

If you'd like some additional help, check out these other resources we offer for your exam:

http://MometrixFlashcards.com/AHIMA

Additional Bonus Material

Due to our efforts to try to keep this book to a manageable length, we've created a link that will give you access to all of your additional bonus material.

Please visit **https://www.mometrix.com/bonus948/rhia** to access the information.